About Bioethics
Philosophical and Theological Approaches

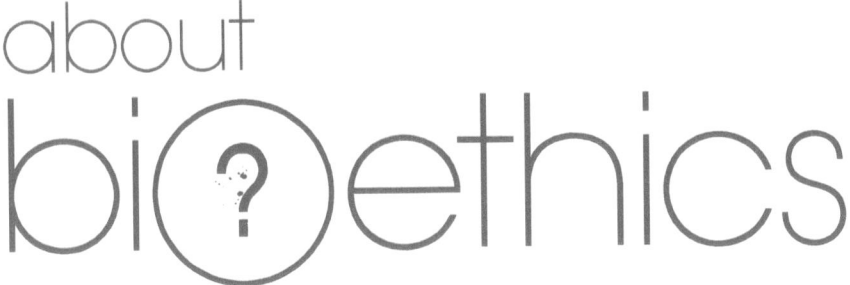

about bi?ethics

PHILOSOPHICAL AND THEOLOGICAL APPROACHES

Nicholas Tonti-Filippini

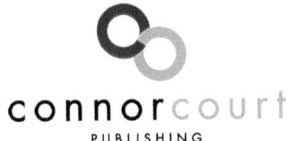

connorcourt
PUBLISHING

Published in 2011 by Connor Court Publishing Pty Ltd.

Copyright © Nicholas Tonti-Filippini, 2011

All rights reserved. No part of this book may be reproduced or transmitted in any form or by any means, electronic or mechanical, including photocopying, recording or by any information storage and retrieval system, without prior permission in writing from the publisher.

Connor Court Publishing Pty Ltd.
PO Box 1
Ballan VIC 3342
sales@connorcourt.com
www.connorcourt.com

ISBN: 9781921421914 (pbk.)

Front cover design: Ian James

Scripture quotations, unless otherwise noted, are from the Revised Standard Version of the Bible.

Excerpts of Vatican documents are from the English translation found on the Vatican webpage: www.vatican.va.

Printed and designed in Australia.

CONTENTS

Preface..1

1. The Culture of Life 9

2. The Foundations of Contemporary Secular Bioethics....17
   - 2.1 Principlism...17
   - 2.2 Liberalism and Autonomy Theory..........................24
   - 2.3 Utilitarian Alternatives...35
   - 2.4 The Contemporary Context of Bioethics................40

3. Theology and the Search for a Universal Ethic..............47
   - 3.1 A Universal Ethic...47
   - 3.2 Written in their Hearts..55
   - 3.3 A Practical Partnership between Faith and Reason...60
   - 3.4 Situation Ethics..69
   - 3.5 Proportionalism and Double-Effect Reasoning.......72
   - 3.6 Fundamental Option...97
   - 3.7 A Natural Law Ethic...100
   - 3.8 Virtue Ethics...114

4. Religion in a Secular Society...123
   - 4.1 Introduction..123
   - 4.2 What is a Secular Society?...................................124
   - 4.3 Public Debate in a Pluralist Society......................126
   - 4.4 State Neutrality about Religion in Australia.........128
   - 4.5 Bigotry about Participation of Religion...............131
   - 4.6 Religious Participation in the Public Square........134
   - 4.7 Secularism and Protecting Religious Freedom.....135

5. **Public Reason and the Case of Bioethics**.....................143

    5.1   A Catholic in a Pluralist Environment.................143
    5.2   The NHMRC Experience..156
    5.3   AHEC's Values in Research....................................158
    5.4   AHEC's Values in Organ and Tissue Transplantation...159
    5.5   AHEC and Care of People Who are Severely Brain Damaged...160
    5.6   AHEC's Moral Language.......................................163

6. **Teaching and Learning Constructive Critical Evaluation**..165

    6.1   Applying the AQF in Bioethics............................165
    6.2   Gatekeepers in Biomedicine..................................166
    6.3   Constructivism is a Natural Outcome...................168
    6.4   Experimenting with Active Learning....................169
    6.5   Developing a Learning Outcome for Constructive Critical Evaluation...................................172
    6.6   Challenges to Constructive Critical Evaluation.....173
    6.7   Problem-based Learning and Constructive Critical Evaluation...178

7. **Bibliography**..183
8. **Index**..193

Preface

The idea for this series came about through illness. For many years I had been teaching and consulting in Bioethics, conducting conferences, publishing articles in the peer reviewed journals, and editing proceedings and the occasional collection, but, apart from writing for the doctorate and masters, I had not ever found time to create a collection of my own work. My time was limited because not only did I have a family, but I have also been chronically ill for thirty-three years with renal disease and have been on haemodialysis for the past twenty years, which is very time-consuming. More recently I developed coronary disease and, following failed bypass surgery, underwent fifteen angioplasty procedures to reconstruct the arteries and place some eight stents to keep them open. The disease has also caused loss of vision and loss of sensation, making typing difficult. It was because I could not travel and because I was ill that this book became possible. Much of the editing was done during dialysis sessions. I am grateful to Vision Australia for the technology, including dictation software, that allows me to keep writing.

In this book I discuss the different approaches to Bioethics both secular and religious and the assumptions and structure of the moral reasoning adopted, the role of religion in a secular society and an approach to teaching Bioethics. This book is to be the first of a series on Bioethics with subsequent books in the series on the Care of the Sick and Dying, Donating Human Organs and Tissue, Man and Woman He Made Them, Motherhood and Technology, Creation, Evolution and the Environment and Protecting the Human Person. The latter is to cover a range of issues such as Experimentation on Human Beings, Capital Punishment, Torture, Identity and Catholic Facilities and Cooperation with Evil.

My interest in Bioethics began in 1977 when, having taken philosophy as a breadth subject, I became interested in it in the same year as I was diagnosed with a rheumatoid disease that was destroying my kidneys and threatening other vital organs. Told that I would die within five years and having become interested in philosophy, I saw no harm in making the latter my principal interest rather than following a more career-oriented path.

Having published in the area of Bioethics, while still a student in 1982, I was asked by Dr Joseph Santamaria, then the Director of Community Medicine at St Vincent's Hospital, Melbourne, and the hospital's Sister Administrator, Sr. Maureen Walters RSC, to assist St Vincent's with the formation of a Bioethics Centre and to assist the director of nursing, Sr Rose Holman RSC, by teaching nursing ethics in the School of Nursing. The position was supported by Dr Joe's brothers, BA Santamaria and John Santamaria, and by Archbishop Sir Frank Little, then archbishop of Melbourne. At the time I was teaching environmental ethics in the Graduate School of Environmental Science at Monash University.

I became hospital ethicist and later Director of the Bioethics Department at St Vincent's while completing graduate studies. I was greatly privileged to work with the Bioethics Centre which then involved Sr Maureen Walters RSC, Sr Rose Holman RSC, Dr John J Billings (of the Ovulation Method), the then dean of the Clinical School, Dr Eric Seal (a psychiatrist), Dr Bernard Clarke (Head of Intensive Care), Rev Dr Francis Harman, Rev Dr Norman Ford SDB, Rev Dr Tom Daly SJ, Rev Dr Laurence Fitzgerald OP and Mr Joseph Santamaria QC, and later Dr Gabrielle McMullen.

Despite never really choosing a career, Bioethics became for me a fulltime occupation.

Working in a hospital with the medical and nursing staff and supported by a group such as that, while battling my own illnesses, was a position of extraordinary advantage for a young person and I am deeply indebted for the opportunities given to me especially by the Sisters of Charity and by Dr Joseph Santamaria. He and the late Dr Francis Harman were my mentors throughout that period. I owe much also to Archbishop Sir Frank Little, who had recommended me to St. Vincent's at a time when I served as a student representative on the Board of Mannix College at Monash University. He took a keen interest, provided some financial support to the Bioethics Centre and made it clear that I was always welcome to call on him. After Mary and I married, he became a visitor to our home in Hawthorn and would often seek an opinion on matters related to Bioethics.

While at St. Vincent's I taught in the School of Nursing, consulted to the medical and nursing staff, and served on numerous medical committees. I also became relatively well known and travelled widely, including many trips to Rome to speak on Bioethics topics. It was an exciting time with the advent of reproductive technology and the development of the document *Donum Vitae* by the Congregation for the Doctrine of the Faith. During that time, Kevin Andrews (later a Minister in the Australian Government) and Anna Duffy (later Krohn) were research officers with the Department at St. Vincent's, and I am grateful for their assistance and for the help of my personal assistant, Mrs Myrna John. I learned much from her and especially through knowing her son Brian, who has Downs Syndrome. Also assisting at that time were several Dominican seminarians, including the future Bishop Anthony Fisher OP and the late Fr Colin Spokes OP, both of whom became great friends. We often pray to Colin asking him to intercede when times are difficult. They both assisted at the St Vincent's Bioethics Centre conferences, carrying the microphones up and down the aisles. At that time I came to know Dr Ray Campbell and Rev Dr John Fleming, with whom I have collaborated many times since.

I met Dr Mary Walsh in November 1982 while attending a Queensland Right to Life conference in Brisbane, having been billeted by a match-making Winifred Egan with Mary and her brother Nicholas. We married in January 1985, having conducted a courtship from afar. Being married to a general practitioner helped me to keep a focus on medical ethics and we formed a team, including undertaking some research on fertility awareness in general practice that resulted in a professional development program based on the Billings Ovulation Method and accredited by the Royal Australian College of General

Practitioners and the Royal Australia and New Zealand College of Obstetrics and Gynaecology. We have been married for twenty-six years and have four children. With my illnesses, Mary has had much to endure, and if I have achieved anything worthwhile it is because she has provided so much love and support, including having given me four children, Claire, Lucianne, Justin and John. My education owes much to them.

In 1990 I was invited by then Monsignor Kevin Manning (later Bishop of Parramatta) to assist him by establishing a Research Office for the Australian Catholic Bishops' Conference. Having moved to Melbourne when we married, Mary graciously moved again with the children for two years to Canberra, and then back again to Melbourne at the end of that time when I went back to work as a consultant, with Archbishop Little as a major client. The two years with the Bishops' Conference was again a time of great privilege, though I can say little about it, still being bound by confidentiality. However I offer the comment that if one likes sausages then one should not see them being made.

At the end of the time with the Bishops I went into end-stage renal failure and it suited me then to be back in Melbourne working as a consultant. The dialysis machine was installed at home and I could combine it with my work. During that time I consulted to the Office of the Australian Prime Minister, UNESCO, the Australian and Victorian Ministers for Health, the Tasmanian Department of State Development, the US Congress and the German Federal Department of Health and Welfare and several hospitals. I also taught in the School of Medicine at Monash University.

In 2001, the John Paul II Institute for Marriage and Family, associated with the Institute of the same name in Rome, opened in Melbourne and I was invited to teach Bioethics and Sexuality there and later took over as head of Bioethics from Rev Dr Anthony Fisher OP when he became an auxiliary bishop to Sydney. I was teaching at the University of Melbourne at the time in the Faculty of Medicine and in the Department of Philosophy.

The Institute is a wonderful place to teach. It is a boutique operation in which we teach Theology, Religious Education and Bioethics to graduate students only, conducting Graduate Diploma, Masters and PhD programs accredited by the Australian Government. Archbishop Denis Hart presides over the Council and has strongly supported the independence of the Institute at a time when the pressure of economies of scale might have produced different results for a small institute such as this. Bishop Anthony Fisher was the founding director and gave the Institute much of its shape and direction. Bishop Peter Elliott is now the Director and the Dean is A/Prof Tracey Rowland. I have known Bishop Elliott for many years, as secretary to Bishop Kelly and later when he was a student at the Institute in Rome. He is much appreciated for his work on the development of religious texts for catholic schools. We have benefitted greatly from his stewardship of the Institute supporting and sustaining the academic life of the Institute while protecting us against the sometimes sharp elbows of life within our very human Church. Tracey has an international reputation as one of the *Communio* group of scholars led by the present Pope Benedict XVI, about whom she has written two books. Others at the Institute who make up our faculty and our discussions include: Dr Adam Cooper, Dr Gerard O'Shea, Dr Colin Patterson, Mrs Anna Krohn and Ms Marcia Riordan. In a way I have come full circle, with the recent introduction of environmental ethics at the Institute, having begun my teaching career on that topic thirty years ago. To assist the Institute, I took an interest in teaching and learning and in 2010 was awarded a Fellowship of the Higher Education Research and Development Society of Australia. I am especially grateful also to Angela Kirsner who edited the text of the book after I had completed it using dictation software, which is far from perfect. I am grateful also for support of our registrar, Colonel Toby Hunter and Promotions Officer, Anthony Coyte.

In recent times I have also served on a number of government committees, including the Australian Health Ethics Committee for two triennia. I was a deputy chair, and chair of several of its working committees, including those on the Unresponsive State and on the Commercialization of Human Tissue. I also served on committees on Assisted Reproductive Technology, Organ and Tissue Transplantation, and Human Research. I am currently a member of an expert panel for the Victorian Assisted Reproductive Technology Authority. It has been a wonderful experience to work in a pluralist context in order to serve the wider community by devising ethical guidelines. I encourage people to join ethics committees. The joint enterprise of seeking to transcend cultural differences and to identify goodness in human relationships is immensely fulfilling.

In 2005, having hosted an international colloquium in Melbourne of the International Association of Catholic Bioethicists, of which I am a member of the governing council, I approached the Australian Catholic Bishops and, with the support of Bishop Christopher Prouse, received approval for an Australian Association of Catholic Bioethicists for which Bishop Anthony Fisher OP is the Episcopal representative. Both associations were formed under the aegis of the Order of Malta, which thus resolved some canonical issues. I am a Knight of Magistral Grace in Obedience in the Order and in 2009, on the gracious advice of Archbishop Denis Hart, Pope Benedict XVI appointed me a Knight Commander of St Gregory the Great for services to Bioethics and the Church. I suspect that Bishop Fisher may have prompted His Grace.

This book contains a range of articles that were published in academic journals, and which have been reworked for this purpose. It also draws on the research and lecture notes for my teaching at the John Paul II Institute, and my earlier teaching in the Faculty of Medicine and the Department of Philosophy at both the University of Melbourne and Monash University. The book is intended to be a guide to Bioethics, discussing the range of different approaches, both philosophical and theological, the engagement between religious and secular Bioethics and an approach to teaching Bioethics. I offer it to students of Bioethics as well as others who have an educated interest in these topics. The books that will follow in the series deal with specific topics in Bioethics including end of life or beginning of life decisions, organ and tissue transplantation, fertility and sexuality.

For me the central concept of Bioethics is respect for every member of the human family. That respect requires us to seek to pursue the good of each one, to avoid the evil of acting in any way that would directly harm each person's flourishing and development, and to respect the role of each in shaping the journey of his or her own life.

Respect for the worth and dignity of each member of the human family has a theological basis in the *imago dei*,[1] but from a purely human perspective, it would be self-defeating to attempt to construct a Bioethic that rejected the notion that every member of the human family has inherent dignity from which we derive each person's equal and inalienable human rights. As a Christian philosopher I am primarily motivated by Christ's instruction that we should love God and one another. That love, so evidenced in His own life, suffering, death and resurrection, also requires us to keep the commandments because their purpose is to protect the good of human development and flourishing. I cannot both love God and love my neighbour and not keep His commandments.

I am deeply in love with Mary, a love that is never static, but which seems to develop in intensity and understanding every day. It is a love that both leads us closer to God and is our witness to His love. Within it we can aim for human perfection despite our weaknesses, and because of it we have been able to cooperate with the Creator in the fruitfulness that is represented in our four children, Claire, Lucianne, Justin and John. They are wonderful evidence of our unity and God's generosity. There is not a day that I do not thank God for all that they give us, the joys, the challenges and above all the purpose of parenting, an overwhelming reason to keep going.

– A/Prof Nicholas Tonti-Filippini
BA (Hons) MA (Monash) PhD (Melb) FHERDSA KCSG
Associate Dean and Head of Bioethics
John Paul II Institute for Marriage and Family, Melbourne

---

[1] Genesis 1 and 2. All biblical quotations are quoted from *The Revised Standard Bible* (London: Collins, 1973).

1

The Culture of Life

The approach that I take to Bioethics is straightforward. It is that every member of the human family possesses inherent dignity and consequently has equal and inalienable rights. I understand inherent dignity to mean that each has intrinsic worth simply by being a member of the human family, no matter their level of maturity or ability and without any other distinction. Being a member of the human family each has the inherent capacity, expressed in their genetic inheritance, of being able to develop as an intellect and to doubt, inquire, wonder and love. Those capacities and our physical nature also mean that we are inherently social beings and it is part of our nature that we live in communion with others. Therefore supporting and protecting human dignity also means fostering and protecting human community. This is what is often called the "culture of life" which is based on the notion of equal and inherent dignity of every member of the human family.

Individuals may express their equal and inherent dignity differently according to their inherited and learned abilities and the choices that each makes within the range of opportunities afforded to them by their life context. There is therefore no single ideal of how to be a good human being. However there are some basic ways in which a person may flourish that are common to all and those basic goods should be encouraged and protected as part of respecting human dignity.

We might begin with protecting each person's own health and life as necessary preconditions for living in human community. Then we can add the pursuit of knowledge of ourselves and the universe and the pursuit of friendship and of family formation and parenthood. This defines what it is to love someone. We love them in supporting their flourishing in each of these ways.

However, as a person of faith, respect for human dignity has a greater context. Each human being is not just a member of the human family with the capacity for intellectual life. That intellectual life has its basis in each being created by God in the Divine image and likeness and each has a vocation to be in communion with the Creator and not just with each other. Human beings are made to love and be loved by the Creator. For a believer, human dignity is not so much anthropocentric but theocentric. Our vocation is to love our neighbours because they too are made in God's image and likeness.

That makes moral goodness straightforward. It is whatever is consistent with seeking to love God and neighbour by fostering and developing that communion of persons for which we were created. Love means seeking to bring about the flourishing of ourselves and others in our universal vocation to seek God's love and the love of neighbour.

That makes moral evil straightforward also. Moral evil means acting in a way that cannot be oriented towards God, including ways that would be contrary to the flourishing of others. Moral evil happens when someone deliberately chooses to destroy a basic good of human flourishing.

In his encyclical *The Gospel of Life,* Pope John Paul II identified that a consequence of our vocation to love God and neighbour is the need to strive for a culture of life. In doing so he contrasted the Gospel message with the culture of death.

The culture of death threatens the most vulnerable in our society: the frail elderly, the chronically ill, those with diminished cognitive function, asylum seekers, the unborn and women who are exposed to the violence of abortion as a solution to what is usually a social problem, the threat of rejection if she accepts her motherhood. In many ways these people are the poorest in our community.

The community of Christ's faithful responds to those threats practically, by our involvement in health care and hospitality, in hospices and palliative care, in assisting asylum seekers, in caring for the sick and the elderly, and by seeking to provide support for women distressed by unexpected pregnancy.

However not only is there a need to give witness by what we offer, there is also a need to influence the development of a culture of life. We need to link our service to the poor, who are the likely victims of the culture of death, with the witness that the Church gives to the dignity of the human person made in the image and likeness of God, a witness that seeks to protect the sacredness of every person but especially the most vulnerable.

Unless we succeed with that witness to the faith, then much of our service to the poor will be undermined by our government, overwhelmed by aggressive secularism, taking away the dignity of those who are most vulnerable. If we do not win the battle for hearts and minds about the sacredness of every human life, then our efforts to serve the poor will become more and more marginalised as the most vulnerable become excluded from membership of the human family.

In seeking to serve the poor, the very basis of that friendship is our acceptance of the fundamental equality of every person. The Order of Malta speaks of "our Lords, the sick." By that we mean to express our role of service to those who are in need of assistance. But this is an obligation for all who share in the love of Christ. True service to the poor does not treat the poor as mere recipients of our beneficence, but fellow travellers along the journey of life. One of the most significant things about volunteering for care of the dying is how often it is that those caring eventually become those cared for.

At heart of the activities of the Church is love for our fellow human beings, and the basis of love is equality. The man who receives my assistance dignifies me by receiving it and I dignify him by recognising my dependence upon him. The mystery of love is its relationship to suffering. Suffering provides the basis for the expression of love. Pope Benedict XVI in his encyclical *Deus Caritas Est* links divine love to human love by showing us that the desire to love someone else is equally a part of complete love as the desire to be loved. *Eros* and *agape* are parts of the same divine love. This is the equality of our love for the poor.

For every woman who is in difficulty with pregnancy there is a man who shares responsibility for the child that is the result of their love. When I stand before an audience of Australian adults, I know that it is likely that one in three persons in the audience has had a direct involvement in abortion. The victims of abortion are all around us. By their lack of love, women and men have harmed themselves through their rejection of the child who is the fruit of their love.

The victims of abortion are part of our spiritual poverty. They are to be numbered amongst our poor to whom we owe service.

Pope John Paul II called for a radical solidarity with women, a solidarity that requires the underlying causes that make a child unwanted to be addressed. There will never be justice, including equality, development and peace, for women or for men, unless there is an unfailing determination to *respect, protect, love and serve life –* every human life, at every stage and in every situation.[2]

Service to this poor is a call to recognise the frailty of human nature and the need for forgiveness. We must ask for forgiveness for ourselves in the choices that we made not to give love where love was needed.

We are called to love practically in service but also in witness to the need of every human being to be loved and respected. The poor, who need what we can give, need also our respect for them as persons, equally called to communion with God our creator.

The attack on that respect for all persons is central to the culture of death, the culture that values human beings only instrumentally for their functions, rather than loving them for who they are. The culture of death is represented by use and not by love. Postmodern secular

---

[2] Pope John Paul II, *Evangelium Vitae*, n. 8. All Vatican documents are cited from http://www.vatican.va.

culture's emphasis on individual narrative and on autonomy excludes all those whose human capacities are diminished.

If we are to provide true service to our Lord's the sick, the frail, the elderly, the cognitively impaired and the other victims of the culture of death, including the victims of abortion, then we must give witness in solidarity with them, calling for recognition of their sacredness and the important role of law in protecting the worth and value of every member of the human family, no matter their disabilities or their loss of dignity through sin.

In the West we face a most difficult battle, one in which as religious persons we are becoming the marginalised. After the second world war, there was a realisation that there was a law above civil law, a set of reasons for human beings to act based upon the inherent dignity and equal and inalienable rights of every human being. For a time there was agreement between the international human rights movement and the great religions.

Since then however we have seen the development of secularism, a very aggressive exclusionist form of secularism, which views religious belief and practice with arrogant intolerance and dismissiveness. This kind of secularist belief is characterised by attempts to exclude contributions to public discussion on the basis of a kind of bigotry that classifies the contributions of persons who are religious in a nominalist way.

The battle has shifted from being a battle about particular issues to a battle in the west for the right of religious persons to exist and to contribute to society in service delivery and to its public policy as religious persons.

When Christians, either as individuals or in company with others of similar mind, take part in public discussion, they do so simply as citizens expressing a view about the common good and the principles that are needed to protect the common good. They are behaving responsibly by taking their civic role seriously, provided of course that they conduct themselves properly within the norms of democracy. This caveat also applies to those who replace intelligent argument and debate with *ad hominem* attacks that invite people to disregard fellow citizens on the basis of their religion.

The view that human life is to be protected is implied by the simple idea of equal respect for persons. It is legitimate to argue about who is a person, but that is not essentially a religious debate, even if religious people may be inclined to be more sensitive to the need to protect those who are most vulnerable, on the fringes of life.

The right to be involved in public debate needs protection. It is manifestly unjust and extraordinarily bigoted to claim that religious people ought not to be permitted to contribute or that their contribution ought not to be considered.

At the same time, contribution to public debate needs to be aware of the sensitivities of others. Public policy advances through seeking points of agreement and being careful to respect areas of disagreement. There is a role for what the philosopher John Rawls calls "public reason"; this is a discussion that takes place on the basis of agreed fundamental principles.

However it is important that there is also continued discussion of those fundamental principles, as well as on the application of them, and it is appropriate in a pluralist society that all perspectives are brought to bear upon that discussion in a considered way.

There is a need to listen to, to search for, and to identify those core values that will make our communities great, whomever and however many espouse them, and from wherever those values might originate.

The great traditions in every age and culture have tended to identify the very same core values. Our human need for a transcendent reality that is beyond the merely human ultimately outlasts every other alternative belief form, both intellectually and emotionally. Every culture has recognised a version of the cardinal virtues:

- *Prudence or wisdom* in recognising and seeking goodness;
- *Temperance* in recognising the need to moderate our desires and inclinations so that they motivate us to serve the good in ourselves and others;

- *Courage* in being able to pursue what we consider to be good;
- *Justice* in recognising the needs of others and the need to give equal respect to all members of the human family.

The community of Christ's faithful has an important role to play in giving witness to those transcendent values. Our role in Bioethics has become a definitive role of leadership in which we defend the poor and their right to be and to exist as fundamental to and in partnership with the practical service that we offer them.

2

The Foundations of Contemporary Bioethics

2.1 Principlism

On July 12, 1974, the National Research Act (Pub. L. 93-348) enacted by the US Congress was signed into law, thereby creating the National Commission for the Protection of Human Subjects of Biomedical and Behavioural Research. One of the charges to the Commission was to identify the basic ethical principles that should underlie the conduct of biomedical and behavioural research involving human subjects and to develop guidelines that should be followed to assure that such research is conducted in accordance with those principles.

The Commission produced what has come to be known as the Belmont report, which defined four principles:[3]

1. **Respect for Persons** – This incorporates at least two ethical convictions and moral requirements: (a) **autonomy:** individuals should be treated as autonomous agents; and (b) **best interests:** persons with diminished autonomy are entitled to protection of their best interests.

2. **Beneficence** – Persons are treated in an ethical manner

---

[3] National Institutes of Health, "Regulations and Ethical Guidelines", http://ohsr.od.nih.gov/guidelines/belmont.html#ethical (accessed August 6, 2010).

not only by respecting their decisions and protecting them from harm, but also by making efforts to secure their well-being. Such treatment falls under the principle of beneficence. The term is often understood to cover acts of kindness or charity that go beyond strict obligation. In this document, beneficence is understood in a stronger sense, as an obligation. Two general rules have been formulated as complementary expressions of beneficent actions in this sense: **(1)** do not harm and **(2)** maximize possible benefits and minimize possible harms. This is often expressed as two principles: **Non-maleficence and Beneficence.**

3. Justice – Who ought to receive the benefits of research and bear its burdens? This is a question of justice, in the sense of "fairness in distribution" or "what is deserved." An injustice occurs when some benefit to which a person is entitled is denied without good reason or when some burden is imposed unduly. Another way of conceiving the principle of justice is that equals ought to be treated equally. However, this statement requires explication. Who is equal and who is unequal? What considerations justify departure from equal distribution? Almost all commentators allow that distinctions based on experience, age, deprivation, competence, merit and position do sometimes constitute criteria justifying differential treatment for certain purposes. It is necessary, then, to explain in what respects people should be treated equally. There are several widely accepted formulations of just ways to distribute burdens and benefits. Each formulation mentions some relevant property on the basis of which burdens and benefits should be distributed. These formulations are: (1) to each person an equal share, (2) to each person according to individual need, (3) to each person according to individual effort, (4) to each person according to societal contribution, and (5) to each person according to merit.

Some have also referred to the four principles as the "Georgetown Mantra" or "Principlism."

In their well-known text on Bioethics,[4] Beauchamp and Childress adopted the four principles as the basis of their analysis of Bioethical issues. They define *principlism* as the idea that ethical justification rests primarily, if not exclusively, in appeals to more general or "higher level" moral norms under which any more particular ethical claim can be subsumed.

Their idea is that the four principles – autonomy, non-maleficence, beneficence and justice – are common to most ethical theories that are applied to Bioethics, so that it does not matter that we approach Bioethics from different perspectives, we hold these principles in common. Beauchamp and Childress seem to have in mind a structure for Bioethics that includes four levels:

- Ethical theories
- Principles
- Rules
- Particular judgements in actual situations.

They claim that their approach follows commonsense, and that it is a top-down bottom-up theory: top-down in that they move from the various theories to the principles, from the principles to the rules, and then apply the rule to particular applications; but then they test and modify the rules and the principles by going from particular cases, and their resolution, to the rules and from the rules to the principles, so that the rules and principles are capable of modification and the approach retains its coherence.

They talk about medical ethics as evolving with the society, from the Hippocratic era, which placed emphasis on non-maleficence and beneficence, to the contemporary era, in which those notions are restrained by respect for autonomy and justice.

Beauchamp and Childress explain that to respect an autonomous agent is, at a minimum, to acknowledge that person's right to hold

---

[4] Tom L. Beauchamp, James F. Childress, *Principles of Biomedical Ethics* (5th Edition) (New York: OUP, 2001).

views, to make choices, and to take actions based on personal values and beliefs. Such respect involves respectful action, not merely a respectful attitude. It also requires more than noninterference in others' personal affairs. It includes, at least in some contexts, obligations to build up or maintain others' capacities for autonomous choice while helping to allay fears and other conditions that destroy or disrupt their autonomous actions. Respect, on this account, involves acknowledging decision-making rights and enabling persons to act autonomously, whereas disrespect for autonomy involves attitudes and actions that ignore, insult, or demean others' rights of autonomy.[5]

Distinctive features of the contemporary era are, they claim, based on recognizing that there is a plurality of viewpoints about the nature of the good to which beneficence may refer and that leads to the autonomy of individuals predominating over any particular theory of the good of human beings. They also refer to widespread cost (profit) consciousness with respect to the application of theories of justice and the imposition of budgetary limits on health care. That then has effects on life-sustaining decisions through the application of measures to assess the worth of health expenditure, such as what are called Quality of Life Years (QALYs). QALYs measure how long a person may live as a result of a procedure and at what quality, which gives a value for a procedure for the purposes of comparison with other procedures in the competition for health funding and the need to ration and manage health care costs.

Beauchamp and Childress claim that society's resources are limited and justice therefore demands that the health care system run efficiently, and also that insufficient resources allocated to health care will lead to an unjust system – balancing efficiency against equity.

They argue that there is ethical justification for a two-tiered system, with equal rights of access to the first tier (a decent minimum standard of health care) and no social subsidies for the second tier, comprising those services that are above the minimum standard. Age, race, gender, social worth are no barriers to first tier access and the fundamental

---

[5] Beauchamp and Childress, op.cit., p. 63.

challenge is to specify the decent minimum in health care. This, they argue, is a social and political decision, and requires regular review and revision of such standards. Once this decent standard is specified, however, patients & physicians must operate by the rules of the two-tier system.

Beauchamp and Childress also acknowledge that compromises to both access and quality of health care can arise from policies of health care organizations, which may only advance business interests alone. There is thus a need for institutional or organizational ethics.

In their system, a just health system will not compromise decent "bedside" quality of health care (including effective communication time); however a just health system does not mean there will be no medically based rationing at "bedside."

Further, educating administrators and accountants about medical ethics is vital so that they can make resource-related health care decisions more validly.

One of the claimed benefits of principlism is that the four principles are commonly held and not dependant on any particular ethical theory. In that way, Beauchamp and Childress claim to be balancing deontology and consequentialism. By deontology is meant ethical theories that lay claim to particular duties towards others. By consequentialism is meant those theories that judge moral actions entirely by the balance of the outcomes.

The weakness of not having an overarching theory for the principles is that there is then no overarching framework from which a judgment could be derived when principles conflict. Beauchamp and Childress address the question of such conflicts in the following way:

> Better reasons can be offered to act on the overriding norm than on the infringed norm... The moral objective justifying the infringement has a realistic prospect of achievement. No morally preferable alternative actions can be substituted. The form of infringement selected is the least possible, commensurate with achieving the primary goal of the action. The agent seeks to

minimize the negative effects of the infringement.[6]

The problems of principlism are that narrowing the real moral problems to certain principles involves some moral reductionism. What we lose is a sense of teleology or overall purpose in health care. In the Hippocratic era the doctor had clear obligations to serve the health needs of the patient. In the modern era that is not so clear, as the obligations are determined by what the patient wants. What the patient wants and what is needed for the patient to develop and flourish are not necessarily the same thing. Having a sense of vocation as a health professional and a set of professional standards may then conflict with the priorities of the individual patient, including objectives that involve using medicine for non-medical ends.

An obvious conflict, therefore, is that between what is called virtue ethics and principlism. The idea of virtue is that a person behaves in ways that are consistent with a character ideal that is itself determined by a teleology. Thus one might say that the aims or teleology of medicine are to prevent or cure disease and disability or a least slow down the progress of disease processes and to manage distressing or uncomfortable symptoms. The virtues that one would expect in a health professional would be those that are determined by those goals, those personal characteristics that would best attain those ends, including those virtues such as respecting confidence, paying attention to the whole person, and respecting the patient's right to refuse intervention, that are part of earning the necessary trust of the patient so that the doctor can serve those goals.

There is a tension between virtue ethics and principlism precisely because principlism has no teleology. There is no objective. That means that there is a tension over the application of the principles, whether they are equal or whether some take precedence. Nowadays the highest principle is autonomy but that excludes a notion of what is good for human beings and is not consistent with a sense of medical vocation.

One area in which principlism seems to fail is in the area of respect

---

[6] Beauchamp and Childress, op.cit., p. 34.

for human life. With the emphasis on autonomy, attitudes to the value of a person's life depends on the value that the individual attaches to his or her own life. That leaves open the issue of the value of the lives of persons who lack autonomy or whose autonomy is reduced by cognitive impairment. It also creates a situation in which respect for a person's life and hence survival depends entirely on that person retaining a will to live. That puts at risk not only those who are cognitively impaired, but also puts at risk those who are seriously or chronically ill and those with disabilities, who may feel that with the option of euthanasia available, they should liberate others from the burden of their care.

Similarly, the emphasis on autonomy removes the sense of medicine only serving legitimate ends. The use of medicine for social purposes, for unnecessary cosmetic surgery and for alternative means of reproduction all become open so long as someone wants medicine for such a purpose, and without regard to what may be the vocational or professional ethical standards of the individual health practitioner or health facility.

Bioethics therefore is much more than principlism. We do need to debate what are the legitimate ends of medicine and important values such as the worth and dignity of every member of the human family and the sacredness of the human body and human relationships. Principlism excludes all such discussion with its emphasis on autonomy and its rejection of any consideration of what is good for human beings. It is inconsistent with a notion of dignity that includes equal respect for persons.

Principlism by its emphasis on autonomy excludes those who are cognitively impaired because it offers no way of recognising human dignity other than as a right to autonomy. By placing the emphasis on autonomy, principlism results in an aggressive and impractical individualism that is not consistent with what it means to be part of a community and the obligations that we each have towards our community. In placing emphasis on individualism, the list ignores the reality that a person with a disability may be largely dependant on his or her family and wider community.

There is an essential inconsistency between the individualism expressed by principlism and the Convention on the Rights of Persons with Disabilities.[7] The preamble to the Convention recognises that disability is an evolving concept and that disability results from the interaction between persons with impairments and attitudinal and environmental barriers that hinders their full and effective participation in society on an equal basis with others.

The crucial notion that is recognised within the field of disability is that the major barriers to participation are not the impairment suffered by the individual but the attitudes of those around them and the failure to provide accessible environments. The major need is for people to remove those barriers to inclusion which often requires the cooperation and goodwill of others. The individualism of the language of "autonomy" misses the point altogether, that representation may be done by someone else and that relationships between a person who has a disability and those who care for them requires communitarianism rather than individualism for all parties.

The emphasis on autonomy also creates difficulties for health care as a vocation. Instead of serving the health needs of patients, health professionals become servants to whatever whim a patient may have.

2.2 Liberalism and Autonomy Theory

Autonomy can be understood as negative or positive freedom.

Negative freedom means that a person or group is or should be left to do what he or she is able to do without interference by other persons, usually qualified by the requirement to the extent that his or her freedom does not impinge upon the equal freedom of others in that respect.

Positive freedom means living in such a way that one is really free, and the promotion of such a life – an issue of character. Positive

---

[7] "Convention on the Rights of People with Disabilities", http://www.un.org/disabilities/convention/conventionfull.shtml (accessed August 6, 2010).

freedom would not include choices that had the effect of restricting a person's freedom such as: selling oneself into slavery, taking drugs that cause addiction or that suppress the cognitive capacity to make competent, informed and free choices, working in situations that endanger life and health and hence future freedom, refusing to be educated because education allows one to be maximally capable of making free choices between alternatives, or refusing to acquire the habit of choosing in a way that seeks to develop the flourishing of oneself and others – something that is necessary to be free, given our embodied nature. Positive freedom is thus related to human flourishing – we are maximally free when we make choices consistent with our flourishing as human beings.

The distinction between negative and positive freedom is made most obvious by the euthanasia debate. Negative freedom demands that people be free to choose suicide or be assisted to suicide. Positive freedom rejects suicide because it ends all human flourishing.

Respect for autonomy therefore is not quite straightforward. Suicide is an autonomous choice to end all future autonomy. Similarly many other "free choices" turn out not to be a choice for freedom, but to limit it – for instance a choice to take a drug of addiction that also suppresses cognitive ability and hence choice, and by being addictive also impeding choice.

Aristotle understood respect for free will (autonomy) as meaning respect for a person because he or she is autonomous (has the ontological status of being a chooser), or more particularly, rationally autonomous, a rational chooser. This is to be distinguished from respecting autonomy in the sense of respecting a person's choices simply because he or she has chosen them. The latter may include choices that would prevent the person from being autonomous such as choices to use an addictive mind altering substance or to commit suicide. The latter view may be called respect for autonomy as a *moral trump*, as the person's own choices for their care over-ride, no matter what they are.

There is some confusion in the literature on autonomy as to which meaning is the more important. Most want to qualify choice and require respect for rational choice rather than mere choice, but that then raises questions as to whose rationality is to apply. If I hold that suicide is irrational because it lacks respect for the person of the chooser, then this view would allow us to override a person's choice to suicide or to use an addictive mind altering substance on the basis that such a choice is not rational because it diminishes or ends their autonomy, their capacity for future choices. There is thus a clash between respecting a person because he or she has free will and is thus autonomous and respecting a person's autonomy as a moral trump. To some extent the euthanasia debate is a contest between these two views of autonomy: respect for the autonomous person or respect for the choices of the autonomous person. As is discussed later, the NHMRC's account of *respect for persons* engages both views in asserting that it means that the individual person has intrinsic worth and it means respect for the values, culture and beliefs of the individual person. However it is obvious that there may be choices that can bring these two perspectives into conflict.

Immanuel Kant had a different view about autonomy, which he contrasted with heteronomy. For him, being autonomous meant acting to a set of norms that were developed through reason free from external influences or one's own upbringing. This was based on his view that "The will is a kind of causality belonging to living beings insofar as they are rational; freedom would be the property of this causality that makes it effective independent of any determination by alien causes."[8]

By this, he meant being free of "impediments to autonomy" such as beliefs that one's behaviour is directed by authority of another or the society or by matters beyond one's control, such as one's genetics, one's nurturing, or the gods or forces of evil. He upheld respect for the role of the will as worth beyond price because governed by the will alone.

---

[8] Immanuel Kant, *The Grounding of the Metaphysics of Morality*, translated by James W. Ellington (Indianapolis: Hackett Publishing Company, 1981), p. 49.

Others have been critical of this as impractical. Barbara Herman held that:

> Autonomy is the condition of the will that makes agency possible. If we were not rational beings, we would not have wills that could be interfered with. But *agency* is not completely described by identifying a will as rational. As human agents we are not distinct from our contingent ends, our culture, our history, or our actual and possible relations to others. Agency is situated. The empirical and contingent conditions of effective agency set the terms of permissibility because it is through effective agency that autonomy is expressed (made real).[9]

Kant is often regarded as the father of modern liberalism and an overriding respect for autonomy. It is therefore important to be clear about what autonomy means for him.

In summary, Kant's notion of autonomy is not:

a) psychological maturity and independence;
b) a moral right;
c) Sartrean autonomy, which lacks commitment to rational principles of a special sort;
d) Rousseau's idea of *moral liberty*, which is more a political notion than a notion about reason and morals;
e) captured by only a distinction between autonomous acts (that is, acts that are rationally willed) and heteronomous acts (acts that are a result of inclination and desire and hence not free).[10]

Thomas Hill maintains instead that Kant's idea of autonomy is:

a) normative rather than metaphysical;
b) to do with reasons and principles for which we act;
c) a property of all adult, sane human beings and inseparable

---

[9] Barbara Herman, *The Practice of Moral Judgement* (Cambridge, Mass.: Harvard University Press, 1993), p. 205.
[10] Thomas E. Hill Jnr, *Dignity and Practical Reason in Kant's Moral Theory* (Ithaca: Cornell University Press, 1992), pp. 77-82.

from "negative freedom;"

d) free in a negative sense, so that an autonomous agent is able to act for the sake of ends other than the satisfaction of desire;

e) not only negative freedom but also freedom "positively conceived."

Another "father of liberalism" is reputed to be John Stuart Mill. Mill is best known in this context for his classical statement of negative freedom:

> ...the sole end for which mankind are warranted, individually or collectively, in interfering with the liberty of action of any other of their number is self-protection. That the only purpose for which power can be rightfully exercised over any member of a civilised community, against his will, is to prevent harm to others. His own good, either physical or moral, is not a sufficient warrant. He cannot rightfully be compelled to do or forbear because it will be better for him to do so, because it will make him happier, because in the opinions of others, to do so would be wise, or even right. These are good reasons for remonstrating with him, or persuading him, or entreating him, but not for compelling him, or visiting him with any evil in case he do otherwise.[11]

However what is interesting about Mill and autonomy is that he argues for it as giving greater value to the person him or herself:

> It is not by wearing down into uniformity all that is individual in themselves, but by cultivating it, and calling it forth, within the limits imposed by the rights and interests of others, that human beings become a noble and beautiful object of contemplation; and as the works partake the character of those who do them, by the same process human life becomes rich, diversified, and animating, furnishing more abundant aliment to high thoughts

---

[11] John Stuart Mill, *Essay on Liberty,* First published in 1859 (Cincinnati, Ohio: Megalodon, 2008), p.13.

and elevating feelings, and strengthening the tie which binds every individual to the race, by making the race infinitely better and worth belonging to. In proportion to the development of his individuality, each person becomes more valuable to himself, and is therefore capable of being more valuable to others.

And further, he argues that autonomy is an intrinsic good:

Having said that the individuality is the same thing with development, and that it is only the cultivation of individuality which produces, or can produce, well-developed human beings, I might here close the argument: for what more or better can be said of any condition of human affairs than that it brings human beings themselves nearer to the best thing they can be? or what worse can be said of any obstruction to good than that it prevents this?[12]

He is not, however, above arguing that autonomy is an instrumental good:

Doubtless, however, these considerations will not suffice to convince those who most need convincing; and it is necessary further to show, that these developed human beings are of some use to the undeveloped - to point out to those who do not desire liberty, and would not avail themselves of it, that they may be in some intelligible manner rewarded for allowing other people to make use of it without hindrance.[13]

Mill is something of an elitist and does not include undeveloped peoples within the defence of autonomy:

For the same reason, we may leave out of consideration those backward states of society in which the race itself may be considered in its nonage. The early difficulties in the way of spontaneous progress are so great, that there is seldom any choice of means of overcoming them; and a ruler full of the spirit of improvement is warranted in the use of any expedients

---

[12] Mill, op. cit., pp. 120-121.
[13] Mill, op. cit., p. 122.

that will attain an end, perhaps otherwise unattainable. Despotism is a legitimate mode of government in dealing with barbarians, provided the end be their improvement, and the means justified by actually effecting that end. Liberty, as a principle, has no application to any state of things anterior to the time when mankind have become capable of being improved by free and equal discussion.

But he also rejects slavery, which would indicate that he is more inclined to support what I have called "positive freedom" rather than negative freedom only. This may have implications for other ways that people may choose to restrict their future autonomy, such as voluntary euthanasia, using drugs of addiction, choices that impair the capacity to make rational choices, or choosing work that endangers life and health, such as prostitution.

Of slavery Mill says;

But by selling himself for a slave, he abdicates his liberty; he foregoes any future use of it beyond that single act. He therefore defeats, in his own case, the very purpose which is the justification for allowing him to dispose of himself. He is no longer free; but is thenceforth in a position which has no longer the presumption in its favour, that would be afforded by his voluntarily remaining in it. The principle of freedom cannot require that he be free not to be free.

He also has a strong view about the obligation to educate children:

Consider, for example, the case of education. Is it not almost a self-evident axiom, that the State would require and compel education, up to a certain standard, of every human being who is born its citizen? Yet who is there that is not afraid to recognise and assert this truth? Hardly anyone indeed will deny that it is one of the most sacred duties of the parents (or, as law and usage now stand, the father), after summoning a human being into the world, to give to that being an education fitting him to perform his part well in life towards others and towards himself. But while this is unanimously declared to be the father's duty, scarcely anybody, in this country, will bear to hear of obliging him to perform it. Instead of his being required to make any exertion or sacrifice for securing education to his child, it is left to his choice to accept it or not when it is provided gratis! It still remains unrecognised, that to bring a child into existence without a fair prospect of being able, not only to provide food for its body, but instruction and training for its mind, is a moral crime, both against the unfortunate offspring and against society; and that if the parent does not fulfil this obligation, the State ought to see it fulfilled, at the charge, as far as possible, of the parent.

The point that I wish to make about respect for autonomy is that it is not clear that respecting autonomy means simply respecting a person's choices. Positive freedom is relevant and may impose limits on what may rightly be chosen and hence respected. Choices that are against the person and their future autonomy may be problematic in areas such as:

- voluntary euthanasia;
- substance abuse;
- voluntary acceptance of paid work in unsafe or unhealthy conditions;
- voluntary acceptance of paid work but without adequate provision for reasonable hours and rest;
- voluntary prostitution;
- voluntary employment as a research subject or as a tissue donor in ways that involve serious harm or grave risk of serious harm.

There is a distinction to be made between respecting human beings because we are rationally autonomous (have free will) and respecting the choices that human beings make. The first is upheld by the Christian tradition. But that respect for the person does not mean that choice confers some kind of validity on an act or a value. True freedom recognises truth and truth includes human development and flourishing. We are not truly free if we act against ourselves. Acts that harm the individual and thus reduce capacity to act freely are acts against freedom. A freedom that claims to be absolute in the sense of absolute respect for choice ends up treating the human body as a raw datum, devoid of any meaning and moral values until freedom has shaped it in accordance with its design. Consequently, in such a scheme human nature and the body appear as *presuppositions or preambles*, materially *necessary* for freedom to make its choice, yet extrinsic to the person, the subject and the human act. The functions of human nature and the human body would not be able to constitute reference points for moral decisions, because the finalities of these inclinations would be merely *"physical"* goods. In this way of thinking, the tension between freedom and a nature conceived of in a reductive way is resolved by a division within man himself.[14]

In medical practice, respect for autonomy means respecting a person's right to refuse treatment that is offered. But it does not extend to a patient being able to direct what treatment is to be offered. Medicine as a vocation seeks to serve genuine medical purposes and according to the evidence as to what is likely to succeed in serving those purposes. Medicine recognizes the reality of human nature and what is needed for a person to flourish. That knowledge informs treatment decisions.

Some useful distinctions can be made between freedom as autarchy, freedom in the sense of being autonomous and freedom in being rationally autonomous. An adult duck on a pond may have *autarchy* in that it is sentient and can live a self-sufficient life, feeding itself without help from others and building its own nesting place.

A gorilla may be *autonomous* in that it is able to make choices, is self governing and not subject to the rules of others, is self aware in a way that a duck may not be, and is able to plan for the future and devise strategies to secure a better future for itself and others.

An adult human being, however, is usually *rationally autonomous* and that means something much more. She is not only self aware but

---

[14] *Veritatis Splendor*, n. 48.

is aware of being self aware and can decide the kind of person, the character that she wants to be. A human being has *dispositional* as well as *occurrent* preferences.[15] By that I mean that she may have an *occurrent* preference for a particular food or some other such immediate liking, but that is different from a *dispositional* preference to be a certain of person, to have an ideal and a preference to live up to that ideal. A human being has a capacity to form a life plan and to undertake the steps necessary, such as education, to achieve that plan. She is also self creative in the sense of recognizing the way she is and effecting deliberate change to be a different type of person. A person who is rationally autonomous acts for rational purposes rather than mere instincts.

The distinctions are important. A person with a severe physical disability, such as quadriplegia, may completely lack autarchy because he or she is so dependant on others for the basic necessities of life, but yet be full rationally autonomous in making his or her own reasoned choices.

There are three types of impediments to rational autonomy: ignorance, coercion, and incomprehension or incompetence.

I may forcibly choose to prevent a person from crossing an unsafe bridge in the belief that he lacks the information that I have that it is unsafe. The lack of information impedes his ability to make the decision that he would have made had he not been ignorant.

I was called to a situation at the hospital where I worked when a patient who was suffering from a burst appendix and in urgent need of surgery decided to leave under the influence of her male relatives. The lady was Moslem and had been brought to hospital by ambulance after collapsing at a supermarket with severe abdominal pain. She was diagnosed with the condition and consented to emergency surgery after having the options explained to her. Later her husband and sons arrived and announced that this was a common and passing occurrence and that she was needed to go home to cook the evening meal. In

---

[15] Robert Young, *Personal Autonomy: Beyond Negative and Positive Liberty* (London: Croome Helm, 1986), pp. 8ff.

their presence she had opted to leave with them. The interpreters had since left and were unavailable, even by telephone. I suggested that the hospital security be called to remove the relatives. When that happened she agreed to continue with the surgery. I judged that in the circumstances her desire to leave was coerced and could be overridden in the first instance, and that was borne out by what happened when the relatives were removed and she was again able to make her own decision.

Similar difficulties can happen with living organ and tissue donation and surrogacy arrangements in which a person may agree under family influence or emotional pressure to decisions that they would not make if given the opportunity to express a view without that pressure. The psychological assessments done for organ donation are designed to discover such difficulties.

Finally, competence can be an issue and may be relative to a particular decision. A patient who had agreed to a hip replacement operation reached the stage of having been pre-medicated prior to surgery on two occasions before refusing on both occasions at the time that she was being moved to the operating room. On both occasions the surgery was not completed much to her desperate frustration and continued pain and disability as she was again placed on the waiting list. I was consulted and suggested what I called a Ulysses contract (after the story of Ulysses and the sirens who, having prevented his men from hearing their song, had himself roped to the mast and forbad the crew to respond to his pleas while they passed the island of the sirens[16]), in which she would agree to her post-premedication wishes being ignored and that she be taken into surgery and operated on despite a refusal at that time. She agreed with the view that the combination of premedication and the proximity of the surgery may have contributed to her state of fear that led her to override her view that she needed and wanted the surgery. In other words, she was temporally incompetent in

---

[16] Clara Erskine Clemet Waters, *A Handbook of Legendary and Mythological Art*, first published in 1875. Available at http://www.archive.org/details/ahandbooklegend-06wategoog (accessed August 6, 2010).

those circumstances with regard to making a rational decision to have the surgery.

Those impediments aside, respect for autonomy in health care is generally understood to mean that the decisions of the patient should be respected and consent is required for treatment except in the circumstances when an emergency renders it not practicable to inform the patient or their representative and obtain consent in time for emergency intervention.

2.3   Utilitarian Alternatives

One of the dominant approaches to Bioethics is called "utilitarianism." Utilitarianism is a form of consequentialism in that decisions are to be based entirely on the predicted outcomes and not on the meaning of human acts. One of the implications of consequentialism is that intentionality, the distinction between acts and omissions, the distinction between intended and merely foreseen consequences and the Pauline principle that one must not do evil in order to achieve good become meaningless. Any connection between affectivity and morality is also excluded, for to act out of love would be to act other than according to the goal of producing the best consequences.

There are varieties of utilitarianism.

Often utilitarianism is presented in terms of hedonism, of seeking pleasure and avoiding pain. It can also be presented in terms of maximizing happiness or in terms of maximizing preference satisfaction.

Hedonism can be explained psychologically on the basis of a claim that pleasure is the only possible ultimate object of desire or pursuit. It can be explained evaluatively in terms of pleasure being what we ought to desire or pursue. Finally, it can be claimed as a rational principle with the claim that pleasure is the only object that makes a pursuit rational.

As a moral theory hedonism can take the form of egoism, the theory that all human actions are motivated by self-interest and in this case the person's own pleasure and avoiding pain. However it can also be a utilitarian theory in which a principle of universalizabilty is applied to egoism, yielding the view that the right action is that which produces the most pleasure (and avoidance of pain) for all (total or average). By universalizability I mean the logical principle that whatever decision I make in a given circumstances, I am committed to making the same decision in like circumstances. It is also variously described in terms of the Golden Rule of Moses that one must do unto others as you would have them do unto you, or in terms of a notion of equality – everyone to count for one and no-one for more than one.

Utilitarianism thus has some appeal as the application of a principle of equality. Its basis in hedonism, however, is questioned because the concepts of pleasure and pain do not quite capture our motivations, even our self-interested motivations.

John Stuart Mill comments in his work *Utilitarianism* wrote: "It is better to be a human being dissatisfied than a pig satisfied; better to be Socrates dissatisfied than a fool satisfied. And if the fool, or the pig, is of a different opinion, it is because they only know their own side of the question. The other party to the comparison knows both sides."

Human happiness is much more complex than simply seeking pleasure and avoiding pain. We will forego the former and accept the latter readily for the sake of a higher goal. Think of a footballer or boxer.

Preference utilitarianism is a response to the oversimplification of hedonistic utilitarianism. In preference utilitarianism an act is obligatory if, and only if, it produces a greater balance of preference satisfaction than any alternative act, giving weight to the relative strength of preferences.

Preference utilitarianism is often presented on the basis of applying a logical requirement of universalizability to preferences such that we must treat other people's prescriptions (desires, preferences) as if they were our own and that if we make a moral judgement about a situation, we must make it about any other relevantly similar situations.[17]

Preference utilitarianism takes it as a given that human beings seek to satisfy their desires or preferences and that universalisability is a rational intuition. That then yields the conclusion, according to preference utilitarians, that we must act according to that set of rules which if adopted universally would produce the greatest balance of preference satisfaction, giving weight to the relative strength of preferences.

An obvious problem with preference utilitarianism relates to the aggregating of preferences and preference satisfaction. Such an aggregation permits great injustice. A preference utilitarian does not uphold a principle of equal respect for persons. If it so happens that the total or average level of preference satisfaction can be attained at the cost of the great suffering of minorities, then the inequality is not considered a problem for the theory by a utilitarian. Yet most of us are concerned about the effect of a policy on the worst-off in society. In fact, the circumstances of the worst-off may be considered a measure of the success of a policy. Utilitarianism may thus be considered to be unjust.[18]

Preference utilitarianism is a desire fulfillment theory. One of the problems with theories of that nature is our intuition or our judgement that not all desires are of equal value. For instance, a person's short-term hunger is not on the same level as their desire to be a good parent or a good teacher or a good doctor. The preference of a tyrant to dominate others does not seem to rank alongside the preference of a Mother Theresa to serve the poor.

Even without interpersonal comparison, we do think that what is best for someone is that that he or she obtain or attain what really is best for them and avoid what is bad for them. We do rank desires

---

[17] This is the structure proposed by R. M. Hare, *Moral Thinking, its Level, Method and Point* (New York: Oxford University Press, 1981).
[18] An argument of this kind is explained by John Rawls, *Political Liberalism* (New York: Columbia University Press, 1996), also in *Justice as Fairness: A Restatement* (Cambridge, Massachusetts: Belknap Press, 2001), a revision of his classic *A Theory of Justice* (New York: Basic Books, 1974).

against objective criteria about values.

In our own lives we also give weight to our longer-term views about the kind of person that we wish to be, and that usually takes precedence over shorter-term desires.[19]

The implications of utilitarianism for medicine are obvious. The individual person counts only as a bearer of preferences. Thus whether someone's life may be taken would depend on whether their continued existence adds to a greater level of preference satisfaction. Those who do not yet have preferences do not enter into the calculation and those with cognitive disabilities do not fare well either for the same reason.

Further, that we live in relationships to one another and are affected by the bonds of love within families has no significance within a utilitarian framework. Thus spending more of one's income on family than on strangers would be a problem, as would donating a kidney to a family member rather than to a more deserving stranger, or saving one's child over others from a burning building.

We do think that motives make a difference. In an example from the literature, elderly Aunt Molly is ill. Nephew Tom visits her and helps her because he loves her. Nephew Bob visits her and helps her because he hopes to be rewarded in her will. Nephew Dave visits her and helps her not because he desires to help but because he believes it is his duty.[20] We evaluate each of their choices differently though acting according to a utilitarian duty would have the same standing as the other examples within a utilitarian schema.

One of the realities of human acts is that as well as external consequences, our acts have an internal meaning. The acts that I perform determine the kind of person that I am. If I deliberately kill someone I make myself a murderer. If I steal, I am a thief. Even if the overall consequences in the circumstances are for the better, those choices still leave me as a murderer or a thief.

There is no doubt that donating money to worthwhile charities

---

[19] Julian Savulescu, "The Present-Aim Theory: A Sub-maximizing Theory of Reasons", *Australasian Journal of Philosophy,* Vol 76, No 2. pp. 229-243.

[20] Norman Bowie and Tom Beauchamp, *Ethical Theory in Business* (Englewood Cliffs: Prentice-Hall, 1979) pp. 16-17.

serving the poor can save lives. By spending money on a new sound system for my home that I could have donated to life-saving charities I have therefore omitted to save lives. According to a utilitarian calculation of the consequences I am as morally responsible for those deaths as though I had killed those people I could have saved.

Most of us however would see a moral difference between the two even if we questioned the consumerism and thought that the money would have been better sent saving lives. There is a distinction between acting and omitting to act. Acting to take someone's life is evil in a way in which omitting to save may not be. Whether I am guilty for having omitted to save life depends on the obligations and the motives. A parent who allows a child to drown in the bath we consider to be culpable. We also consider motive. A person who allows someone to drown in order to inherit after their death may be considered to be as culpable as they would be if they actually killed for the same reason.

However the simplicity of utilitarianism, in which the meaning of a decision is not at issue, just the predicted consequences, leaves no place to consider the nature of personal obligation or motive.

Pope John Paul presented the anatomy of a moral act in terms of both the end or intended consequences and the means. An act can be evil because the bad consequences outweigh the good consequences, but it can also be evil if the means is evil or because the intended consequence or goal of the activity is evil.[21,22]

This is discussed in the following chapter, "A Search for a Universal Ethic." The teaching differs from utilitarianism and consequentialism in general because it accepts that an act can have a meaning that renders it intrinsically evil such that no balance of consequences could justify it. This is the meaning of the Decalogue in which God has given us a list of types of act which always are contrary to love because they involve the destruction of a basic human good or failure to fulfil an obligation towards a basic human good.

---

[21] *Veritatis Splendor*, n. 72.
[22] *Veritatis Splendor*, n. 78.

2.4 The Contemporary Context of Bioethics

The Hippocratic tradition really came to an end in the early part of the twentieth century when the Hippocratic oath ceased to be required for graduates of most medical colleges. Around that time we saw the birth of movements to promote euthanasia and eugenics. The issue of euthanasia did not gain much traction except perhaps in Germany, but the eugenics movement more or less became part of the science of medicine.

Some significant events that indicated the acceptance of eugenics were:

- The case of the *Willowbrook State School* in New York City in which children with developmental disabilities were deliberately infected with hepatitis as part of a research project into the effects of gamma globulin. The parents reportedly agreed in exchange for gaining admission for their children. The school was designed for 4,000 and had a population of 6,000 in 1965. At the time it was the biggest state run institution for the "mentally retarded" in the United States.[23]
- Prisoners and people who were mentally ill in asylums were used for harmful research. For instance in the US both prisoners and the inmates of asylums were given X-ray therapy as an experimental treatment for head-lice, and others were deliberately infected with malaria to test the efficacy of drug treatment, which also had significant side effects.[24]
- Eugenics laws were passed in many western countries. California law permitted the forcible sterilization of over 20,000 mentally disabled men and women between 1909

---

[23] Geraldo Rivera, *Willowbrook: A Report on How It Is and Why It Doesn't Have to Be That Way* (New York: Random House, 1972).

[24] Nathaniel Comfort, "The prisoner as model organism: malaria research at Stateville Penitentiary" *Studies in History and Philosophy of Biological and Biomedical Sciences* Vol 40, No. 3, September 2009, pp. 190-203.

and 1970. Similar provisions existed in other States. In the United Kingdom, the 1913 *Mental Deficiency Act* permitted compulsory sterilisation of those in mental asylums.

In the period before the 1913 *Mental Deficiency Act* was introduced in the UK by Sir Winston Churchill's successor as Home Secretary, Churchill, then Home Secretary, wrote in a letter to Lord Asquith: "The unnatural and increasingly rapid growth of the feeble-minded classes, coupled with a steady restriction among all the thrifty, energetic and superior stocks constitute a race danger which it is impossible to exaggerate. I feel that the sources from which the stream of madness is fed should be cut off and sealed up before another year has passed."[25]

When the Mental Deficiency Bill was finally introduced in 1912, in urging its passage, Churchill's successor as Home Secretary, Reginald McKenna, said: "I commend it to the House in the confident assurance that if it is passed into law we shall be taking a great step towards removing one of the worst evils in our time."[26]

Between 24 and 30 July 1912, a month after the Second Reading of the Mental Deficiency Bill in Parliament, the first international Eugenics Conference was held in London, and was attended by four hundred delegates. Churchill was a Vice-President of the Congress, and Alexander Graham Bell, the inventor of the telephone, was one of its directors, as was Charles Eliot, a former President of Harvard, and the Regius Professor of Medicine at Oxford, Sir William Osler. The Canadian-born Osler, who had been created a baronet the previous year, was one of the world's most prominent practitioners of clinical medicine. The Congress opened with a reception and a banquet that was addressed by the former Prime Minister, A.J. Balfour.[27]

We often attribute the eugenics movement to Nazi Germany but it is clear that, before the Second World War, many of the eugenic attitudes and practices that were later condemned were widespread throughout

---

[25] Letter from Sir Winston Churchill to Lord Asquith, December 1910, http://www.winstonchurchill.org/support/the-churchill-centre/publications/finest-hour-online/594-churchill-and-eugenics (accessed August 6, 2010).
[26] Letter from Sir Winston Churchill to Lord Asquith, op. cit.
[27] Letter from Sir Winston Churchill to Lord Asquith, op. cit.

the western world. With the end of that war came the realization of the extent of the barbarity that had been lawfully practised.

The use of euthanasia during the Nazi era developed as a result of laws being passed to permit it on eugenic grounds. The death ovens later used for genocide had their origins in the extermination of those with developmental disabilities. *Aktion T 4,* the Nazi euthanasia program to eliminate "life unworthy of life," at first focused on newborns and very young children. Midwives and doctors were required to register children up to age three who showed symptoms of mental retardation, physical deformity, or other symptoms included on a questionnaire from the Reich Health Ministry. The Nazi euthanasia program quickly expanded to include older disabled children and adults. Hitler's decree of October, 1939, typed on his personal stationery and back-dated to September 1, enlarged "the authority of certain physicians to be designated by name in such manner that persons who, according to human judgment, are incurable can, upon a most careful diagnosis of their condition of sickness, be accorded a mercy death." The letter to Reishsleiter Bouhler and Dr. med. Brandt, signed by Hitler, instructed them to broaden the powers of physicians designated by name, who would decide whether those who had – as far as could be humanly determined – incurable illnesses could, after the most careful evaluation, be granted a mercy death. According to Milton Meltzer, between December 1939 and August 1941, about 50,000 to 60,000 German children and adults were secretly killed by lethal injection or in gassing installations designed to look like shower stalls. It was a foretaste of Auschwitz. The victims were taken from the medical institution and put to death.[28]

Asked during his trial at Nuremberg, What was Hitler's idea of enthanasia? What did he understand by it? Brandt responded, "The decisive thing for him was also expressed here in the decree, namely, that incurably sick persons – actually it should have read insane persons – other persons were absolute exceptions – could be accorded

---

[28] "Hitler was a Leftist: Hitler's Euthanasia Initiative", http://constitutionalistnc.tripod.com/hitler-leftist/id16.html (accessed August 6, 2010).

a mercy death. That is, therefore, a measure dictated by purely humane considerations, and nothing else could be thought under any circumstances, and nothing else was ever said to me."[29]

On 13th January 1941, the first transport of mentally sick and disabled persons arrived from the psychiatric hospital Eichberg at the newly established killing centre Hadamar near Limburg. After a few hours, the patients were killed by gas and their remains were burnt in the crematorium. Until August of the same year, more than 10,000 people were killed in the gas chamber of Hadamar.[30]

After the war, the Nuremburg trials proceeded on the basis that there is a law above the civil law. The law used to prosecute the Nazi doctors defined as a criminal offence, atrocities and offences, including but not limited to murder, extermination, enslavement, deportation, imprisonment, torture, rape, or other inhumane acts committed against any civilian population, or persecutions on political, racial or religious grounds *whether or not in violation of the domestic laws of the country where perpetrated*.[31] Only in that way could the lawful activity of the doctors be prosecuted as crimes. They were crimes against humanity that a reasonable person should have recognized as crime no matter what the civil law permitted.

The reactions to the atrocities saw the development of the international human rights movement led by Dr Eleanor Roosevelt in 1949, and the foundation principle expressed in the preambles of the several of the documents that every member of the human family has inherent dignity and equal and inalienable rights, and that that inherent

---

[29] "The Nikzor Project: Extracts from the testimony of Karl Brandt", http://www.nizkor.org/ftp.cgi/places/ftp.py?places//germany/euthanasia/brandt.001, (accessed August 6, 2010).
[30] "The 'euthanasia' crime in Hadamar", http://www.chgs.umn.edu/histories/documentary/hadamar/the_occurrence.html (accessed August 6, 2010).
[31] "Control Council Law No. 10, Punishment of Persons Guilty of War Crimes, Crimes Against Peace and Against Humanity," December 20, 1945, 3 *Official Gazette Control Council for Germany* 50-55 (1946), http://www1.umn.edu/humanrts/instree/ccno10.htm, (accessed August 6, 2010).

dignity is the basis of all rights.[32]

That international acceptance of a universal ethic that transcends cultural and religious boundaries and is above positive law was short-lived. In the post-modern era, individualism has reduced moral discussion to individual narratives and the rejection of objective moral norms. The international human rights movement appears to have been a short blip in the enlightenment project and we are back with the same reductionism and reliance on positivism that spawned the atrocities of the Nazi era. There are still appeals to the need for human rights and countries that do not have a bill of rights are regarded as failing in their obligations to the human rights movement. But what is now meant by rights no longer has a basis in human dignity incorporating equal respect for each member of the human family as an individual of inestimable worth no matter his or her level of ability. Rather, the basis of rights in this era tends to be respect for autonomy in which individual choice alone confers legitimacy. That then sees emphasis being placed on the politics of inclusion with respect to an issue such as same-sex marriage or access by single people to reproductive technology, for instance, despite the emphasis in the instruments on the rights of children based on their need for an identity and to be nurtured by their natural parents and to have access to both their mother and their father, and based also on the role of the State in marriage, because marriage is an institution that protects the interests and security of children.

In this post-modern era there are significant barriers to moral discussion and the social development of public morality. We encounter moral discussion-stoppers such as the following claims:

- We are a pluralist society so people disagree on solutions to moral issues and there is no right or wrong answer.
- Who am I to judge others?
- Morality is a private matter.
- Morality is simply a matter for individual cultures to decide.

---

[32] "Preambles of the International Covenant on Civil and Political Rights and the International Covenants on Economic, Social and Cultural Rights", http://www2.ohchr.org/english/law, (accessed August 6, 2010).

In response to the claim that people disagree on solutions to moral issues, it may be acknowledged that experts in many areas disagree on key issues in their fields. The search for knowledge does not always yield uniformity, but that does not mean that there is no truth, just different understanding of the truth and different pathways for discovering and recognizing truth. There are also many moral issues on which people agree. There are values that transcend or are common across cultures and religions, such as those contained in the international human rights instruments. Disagreements may be about non-moral facts of the matter, about the priorities of values, or even about agreement to participate in a common project of seeking a public morality. Despite the disagreements, the process of public policy formation does involve choosing one morality rather than others. How we protect those unable to choose for themselves involves decisions about their worth and about what is good for them.

The response to "who am I to judge others?" is that deciding whether something is the right course of action is not the same thing as judging a person. There is a distinction between judging as condemning and judging as evaluating. Some forms of judgement are necessary, such as who should be delegated to a task, employed or sacked. Also important, however, is for us to discuss the morality of human acts and, in the professions, what goals are shared in common and what professional virtues are necessary for those professional goals to be achieved.

Morality is not a private matter because sharing common purposes and thus a common morality is what establishes and to an extent defines a community. Some aspects of morality are thus essentially public. Being able to discuss and to reason about morality is important and allows us to recognize the harm that our choices may cause.

Moral choices are not isolated personal preferences, but are to do with interpersonal relationships and living in community.

Nor is morality simply a matter for individual cultures to decide. There is an important distinction between describing a morality and adopting a morality. There are moral principles that transcend culture because they are based on shared human reality, and on that basis we need to be able to discern whether a cultural practice should be changed, such as the cultural practice of female genital mutilation, for instance, or the practice of capital punishment.

3

The Search for a Universal Ethic

3.1 A Universal Ethic

In 2009, the International Theological Commission, with the approval of the President of the Congregation for the Doctrine of the Faith, Cardinal William J. Levada, published *The Search for Universal Ethics: a New Look at Natural Law*.

Amongst other matters, the document discusses the exchange on the level of reason about what is common to all men endowed with reason, and the requirements for establishing a just society.

In Western society, we are witnessing the growth of a secularism that has not only discarded Christianity, but also the balance between God, man and nature that, is at the heart of our tradition, and with it, the teleology that gives meaning and purpose to human activity. In its place is an individualism that in this post-modern era rejects principled conduct in favour of life lived as an individual narrative, judged only for its autonomy.

The Commission's paper has much to offer those of us who must resolve the very practical matter of how to conduct oneself as a Catholic bioethicist, philosopher or theologian in the public forum in which much of Bioethics is conducted. The Commission cautions us to "be modest and prudent when invoking the evidentness of the precepts of the natural law", but nonetheless calls on us to engage in a dialogue with a view to a universal ethic.[33]

The Commission refers to the convergence of philosophy and religion in the natural law[34] and goes on to say that the doctrine of natural law possesses coherence and validity on the philosophical plane of reason common to everyone, but acquires its full sense within the history of salvation: in fact Jesus Christ, sent by the Father, is, with his Spirit, the fullness of every law.

The Commission also explains the dependence of the natural law on grace:

> Grace does not destroy nature but heals it, strengthens it, and leads it to its full realization. For this reason, even if the natural law is an expression of reason common to all men and can be presented in a coherent and true manner on the philosophical level, it is not external to the order of grace. Its claims are present and operating in the different theological states through which our one humanity has passed in the history of salvation.[35]

However, the society that we confront insists on a rigid separation between religious belief and the formation of public policy. In response, many Catholic bioethicists seek to engage in public debate as though natural law can be developed as a matter of pure reason as a discussion about humanity alone, and on such grounds seek to win support for a natural law approach without expecting an audience to listen to claims made from a faith perspective.

It seems to me that, as a matter of recent history, that approach is a failure. The UK probably provides the clearest example of a concerted effort by Catholic intellectuals to take that approach, and the UK probably leads the way in the Western world in terms of adopting evil public policies that are aggressively bigoted in the active exclusion of religious views and of natural law concepts, particularly the rejection of the Pauline principle and moral absolutes that are at the core of

---

[33] International Theological Commission, "The Search for a Universal Ethic 2009", n. 52. There is no official English version available. However an English translation by Joseph Bolin, March 9, 2010 is available at www.pathsoflove.com/universal-ethics-natural-law.html. The official French and Italian versions are available at http://www.vatican.va/roman_curia/congregations/cfaith/cti_index.htm, (accessed August 6, 2010).
[34] "The Search for a Universal Ethic", op. cit., n.11.
[35] "The Search for a Universal Ethic", op. cit., n. 101.

natural law explanations. UK public policy also rejects any notion of sexual ethics other than that there be consent.

Such an approach to secular discussion sells us short by leaving out important elements, such as the theological virtues, and what we know of human and divine love and the communion of persons revealed in the person of Christ and in the Blessed Trinity. St Thomas taught that the theological virtues are not derived from reason but from revelation. To proceed in these debates without those Christian presuppositions robs us of much that is important to understanding our moral tradition, including, I argue, an understanding of moral absolutes and the Pauline principle.

From a Catholic perspective, what we have to offer is an alternative approach to philosophical analysis that constructively builds upon shared understanding, mutually seeking the transcendent. In that ,we can accept the different cultures within our pluralistic society as raw data and can work to identify goodness as a common ground and knowable. That then permits us, in a culturally inclusive way, to transcend differences between religions and cultures while still founded upon those differences. That approach is especially open to the Christian notion of love, asking simply that it be considered as an alternative and asking the very practical question whether a civilisation based on a notion of love as gift of self is a better civilisation than the alternatives.

Basically I am claiming that Christian philosophy has much to contribute to Bioethics from a tradition of exploration of human nature and identifying doctrines that are good for mankind and justified in human terms. As a Christian philosopher I am formed by faith but willing to test its propositions, knowing that God loves us and wants what is good for us. The propositions of the natural law are testable for validity and consistency even if the rich content is to a significant extent dependant on faith and grace.

In 2009, the Congregation for the Doctrine of the Faith also released the document *Dignitas Personae*, which identified three major issues involved in reproductive technology:

a) the right to life and to physical integrity of every human being from conception to natural death;

b) the unity of marriage, which means reciprocal respect for the right within marriage to become a father or mother only together with the other spouse;

c) the specifically human values of sexuality which require "that the procreation of a human person be brought about as the fruit of the conjugal act specific to the love between spouses."

As a faithful Catholic bioethicist, one is inclined to ask, how might these principles be proposed and explained to our contemporary culture as part of a universal ethic? The Congregation envisages that reason and faith are not mutually exclusive, but support each other and intersect, but it also claims that these norms are inscribed in nature and thus available. In defense of the first principle, the Congregation asserts:

> The respect for the individual human being, which reason requires, is further enhanced and strengthened in the light of these truths of faith: thus, we see that there is no contradiction between the affirmation of the dignity and the affirmation of the sacredness of human life. 'The different ways in which God, acting in history, cares for the world and for mankind are not mutually exclusive; on the contrary, they support each other and intersect. They have their origin and goal in the eternal, wise and loving counsel whereby God predestines men and women 'to be conformed to the image of his Son' (*Rom* 8:29).'[36]
>
> By becoming one of us, the Son makes it possible for us to become "sons of God" (*Jn* 1:12), "sharers in the divine nature" (*2 Pet* 1:4). This new dimension does not conflict with the dignity of the creature which everyone can recognize by the use of reason, but elevates it into a wider horizon of life which is proper to God, giving us the ability to reflect more profoundly on human life and on the acts by which it is brought into existence.[37]

In defence of the principles with respect to procreation, the Congregation asserts:

> Natural law, which is at the root of the recognition of true equality

---

[36] "The Search for a Universal Ethic", op. cit., n. 8.
[37] "The Search for a Universal Ethic", op. cit., n. 7.

between persons and peoples, deserves to be recognized as the source that inspires the relationship between the spouses in their responsibility for begetting new children. The transmission of life is inscribed in nature and its laws stand as an unwritten norm to which all must refer.[38]

Attempting to address topics such as those posed within reproductive technology about respect for human life and about procreation and even more widely on matters such as the recognition of homosexual relationships, we are at the same time confronted by a culture that wants to separate humanity from nature. The Commission expresses it as a rejection of the balance between God, man and nature that is at the heart of our tradition.

Gradually as laws are written to deal with the new technologies, the biological realities of human procreation are becoming ignored. In my own home state of Victoria in Australia, fatherhood has been removed from the law altogether. There are mothers identified as those who give birth, and then there are parents and a child may have any number of people who consent to being nominated as "parents" by the birth mother. In this way the law can cope with the myriad possibilities for family formation by removing altogether the significance of the biology of conception, and can adapt to the possibilities including that two men may parent a child by engaging a woman to carry the child for them (using gametes from any source), and then have her name them as the child's parents.

How, in such a cultural context can one defend the balance between God, man and nature that is at the heart of our tradition? Is philosophy enough?

The present Pope, then Professor of Theology at the University of Regensburg, wrote a critique of the treatment of the relationship between philosophy and theology in the Second Vatican Council document *Gaudium et Spes*. He referred to there not being a radical enough rejection of a doctrine of man divided into philosophy and theology, and the tendency for a schematic representation of nature

---

[38] *Dignitas Personae*, n. 6.

and the supernatural being merely juxtaposed.[39]

Presumably he had in mind teachings such as:

> This Sacred Synod, therefore, recalling the teaching of the first Vatican Council, declares that there are "two orders of knowledge" which are distinct, namely faith and reason; and that the Church does not forbid that "the human arts and disciplines use their own principles and their proper method, each in its own domain;" therefore "acknowledging this just liberty," this Sacred Synod affirms the legitimate autonomy of human culture and especially of the sciences.[40]

The approach in *Gaudium et Spes* to philosophy and theology that particularly seems to merely juxtapose faith and reason is also evident in the following passage (GS n. 62):

> Although the Church has contributed much to the development of culture, experience shows that, for circumstantial reasons, it is sometimes difficult to harmonize culture with Christian teaching. These difficulties do not necessarily harm the life of faith, rather they can stimulate the mind to a deeper and more accurate understanding of the faith. The recent studies and findings of science, history and philosophy raise new questions which affect life and which demand new theological investigations. Furthermore, theologians, within the requirements and methods proper to theology, are invited to seek continually for more suitable ways of communicating doctrine to the men of their times; for the deposit of Faith or the truths are one thing and the manner in which they are enunciated, in the same meaning and understanding, is another.

Cardinal Ratzinger also described as a fictional starting point the claim that it is possible to construct a rational philosophical picture

---

[39] Joseph Ratzinger, "The Dignity of the Human Person" in Herbert Vorgrimler (ed) *Commentary on the Documents of Vatican II*, Volume V, (London: Burns & Oates, 1969) pp. 115-163. I am grateful to my colleague Tracey Rowland for identifying the quotations from Cardinal Ratzinger.

[40] *Gaudium et Spes*, n. 59.

of man intelligible to all and on which all men of goodwill can agree, "the actual Christian doctrines being added to this as a sort of crowning conclusion."[41]

In this he would seem to have challenged the presupposition of the Commission that there can be a universal ethic.

In the same article, Ratzinger was highly critical of the Thomists, saying that it can hardly be disputed that as a consequence of the division between philosophy and theology established by the Thomists, a juxtaposition has gradually been established which no longer appears adequate. "There is, and must be, a human reason *in* faith, yet conversely, every human reason is conditioned by historical standpoint so that reason pure and simple does not exist."[42] It should be noted that a debate rages among Thomists over whether a philosophical model or a more Augustinian Thomism properly represents St Thomas.[43] There would seem to be Thomists on both sides of that debate. The debate has significance for the way in which we approach public policy formation. If all that needs to be said about public policy could be developed as a matter of pure reason, we would have no need to bring our faith into the issue of public policy but could debate the issues purely on the basis of reason. But is reason sufficient for that purpose? The International Theological Commission's caution about being modest and prudent when invoking the evidentness of the precepts of the natural law would seem to be relevant.[44] In my experience, many people do not find the precepts of the natural law to be self-evident. Our starting point needs to be somewhere else. Perhaps the least accepted precept of the natural law is the Pauline principle. Many people, it seems, are prepared to do the lesser evil to achieve better consequences.

---

[41] Ibid.
[42] Ibid.
[43] I am grateful to my colleague Tracey Rowland for drawing my attention to the Thomists' differences of opinion. I read with interest the contributions to Volume 83, Summer 2009, No.3 of the *American Catholic Philosophical Quarterly*, which was devoted to a discussion of contemporary Thomisms.
[44] International Theological Commission, op. cit., n 52.

The Pauline principle is explicable within the context of understanding what it is to act in a way that is incapable of being oriented towards God. In the Sermon on the Mount Jesus makes a distinction between his account of the Decalogue and his account of the Beatitudes. The first captures the gravity of the law. The second explains the lesser importance but nevertheless significance of what is demanded by love. In his encounter with the rich young man, Jesus makes a similar distinction between keeping the law in order to be good, but if one is to be perfect then the Beatitudes apply. In doing evil by acting in breach of the law, we sever the relationship with God, and no achievement of good consequences can balance that. The problem in a secular context is how to explain the gravity of doing evil without reference to our relationship to God.

Sitting on government committees drafting ethical guidelines, I discovered that there was a natural desire to distinguish between the words "must" and "should." In drafting guidelines, the committees wanted to describe some guidelines as exceptionless, whereas other principles were not held to be so, although it was difficult to provide a coherent reasoned explanation of the basis for this distinction.

Trying to explain moral norms without recourse to faith is often difficult and in some circumstances may not be possible for a contemporary audience. Cardinal Ratzinger's view in that respect would also seem to be reflected in *Dignitas Personae* (n.7) which, quoting John Paul II in *Veritatis Splendor* (n. 45) states:

> The respect for the individual human being, which reason requires, is further enhanced and strengthened in the light of these truths of faith: thus, we see that there is no contradiction between the affirmation of the dignity and the affirmation of the sacredness of human life. "The different ways in which God, acting in history, cares for the world and for mankind are not mutually exclusive; on the contrary, they support each other and intersect. They have their origin and goal in the eternal, wise and loving counsel whereby God predestines men and women "to be conformed to the image of his Son" (*Rom* 8:29).[45]

---

[45] *Dignitas Personae*, n. 7.

3.2 Written in their Hearts

The issue of the role of reason as distinct from faith with respect to the natural law is reflected in the debate over what is sometimes disparagingly called the "Hellenization of the early tradition,"[46] which may also be attributed to the influence of St Paul, with his background and philosophical education as a Roman citizen, and the Hellenic influences on Roman culture. In relation to natural law, the scriptural text most often quoted is St Paul's letter to the Romans:

> When Gentiles, who do not have the law, do instinctively things required by the law, they are a law for themselves, even though they do not have the law, since they show that the requirements of the law are written on their hearts, to which their conscience also bears witness, and their conflicting thoughts will accuse or perhaps excuse them on the day when, according to my gospel, God, through Jesus Christ, will judge the secret thoughts of all.[47]

St Paul's attitude to philosophy is confusing. He is negative about philosophy but evidently used the language of philosophy of the period and locality in which the Stoics had much influence. He would have been familiar with Aristotle, of whose works the Stoics made free use. His reasoning reflects Aristotle, of an earlier period, and Stoics of the day – Seneca, Epictetus, Marcus Aurelius and Cicero.

Historically St Paul would have had a Greek philosophical training as a Roman citizen and clearly used Stoic arguments. He clearly believed that knowledge can be attained through reason and that ethics is constituted by knowledge. That is to say, he was a cognitivist. In relation to the Stoic naturalist ethics of the period, it is worth mentioning that the Stoics adopted the cardinal virtues (wisdom, justice, courage and temperance) and believed in the inherent goodness

---
[46] This is discussed by Joseph Cardinal Ratzinger in "Faith, Religion and Culture" in *Truth and Tolerance* (San Francisco; Ignatius Press, 2004), pp. 90-95, in which he argues that there is simply a congruence of Greek philosophy and Biblical themes that had in any case occurred before Christ.
[47] Romans 2:14-16.

and purposefulness of human nature, and that the end of human beings was in community. St Paul would not have shared their belief that all people are manifestations of the one universal spirit (pantheism), but he clearly had adopted the view that the Stoics share with Christ that we should live in brotherly love and readily help one another.[48]

In his interesting account of the influence of Stoic philosophy on St Paul, Troels Engber-Perdersen suggests that St Paul adopts the same logic and simply substitutes *Christ* for *Reason* in explaining righteousness in terms of love and communio.[49]

Comparing St Paul to the Stoics, they both claim that goodness is knowable. For the Stoics that is through reason, but for St Paul it is through Christ (Gal 1:16, 2Cor 4:6). In *Corinthians* he makes the revealing comment: "Jews demand signs, Greeks desire wisdom but we proclaim Christ crucified" (1Cor 1:22-25). Also in the same letter he seems to embrace communitarianism using language of the Stoics (1 Cor 1:10-11) and elsewhere he shares the dominance of will and reason over pain and suffering (Gal 5:24) and concludes that joy is the proper response to suffering (Phil 2:17, 1:17-18), both Stoic claims.[50]

St Paul had of course been a Pharisee and trained under the major Jewish scholar Gamaliel (*Acts* 22:3) but his teaching in relation to Pharisaic Law seems to differ depending on the audience. He addresses Gentiles, Jews and Greeks differently. The dominant motif in his teaching is, of course, not reason, natural law or Pharisaic Law, but the Christ event. This is most evident in *Galatians*, and he claims authority on the basis of his "meeting" with Christ on the Road to Damascus.

In relation to claims about the Hellenization of Christianity through St Paul, it is worth noting that Pope John Paul II says something that reinforces this view in his analysis of two difficult passages.

---

[48] Joseph A. Fitzmeyer SJ, *Paul and his Theology: A Brief Sketch* (New Jersey: Prentice Hall,1989) pp. 27-34; *see* also Troels Engber-Perdersen, *Paul and the Stoics* (Edinburgh: T&T Clark, 2000).
[49] Troels Engber-Perdersen, op. cit.
[50] Ibid.

In the very familiar submission and headship passage of *1 Corinthians* (11:2-16), St Paul asserts that Christ is the head of every man, man is head of woman, and also that man is image of God's glory but woman is a reflection of man's glory, as woman came from him. He says also that man is not created for the sake of woman, but woman is created for the sake of man. In his analysis of this passage and the related passage in *Ephesians*, Pope John Paul II asserts:

> The motif of "head" and of "body" is not of biblical derivation, but is probably Hellenistic [Stoic?]. In Ephesians this theme is utilized in the context of marriage (while in First Corinthians the theme of the "body" serves to demonstrate the order which reigns in society). From the biblical point of view the introduction of this motif is an absolute novelty.[51]

Developing the submission and headship theme in Ephesians 5: 22-33, St Paul writes that husband and wife should defer to one another in obedience to Christ, and that wives should regard their husbands as they regard the Lord: Christ is head of the Church and saves the whole body, so is husband head of his wife. Just as the Church submits to Christ, wives submit to their husbands. Husbands should love their wives as Christ loved the Church and sacrificed himself for her.

On this passage Pope John Paul II writes in *Mulieres Dignitatem* (n. 24) that St Paul was rooted in the customs of the time. Adapting the teaching, the Pope writes that there should be mutual subjection out of reverence for Christ, and that the husband is "head" in order to give himself up for his wife. The Pope asserts that "subjection" is not one-sided but mutual. I mentioned these treatments of St Paul by Pope John Paul II to a Pauline Conference[52] recently and was greeted by what can only be regarded as a seething response by a recent convert from Lutheranism.

---

[51] Pope John Paul II, *The Theology of the Body: Human Love in the Divine Plan* (Boston: Pauline Books & Media, 1997), p. 382.
[52] *A Pauline Colloquium* conducted by the John Paul II Institute for Marriage and Family, Melbourne July 27-8, 2007.

What is clear about St Paul's treatment of Pharisaic Law is that he adapts to particular audiences but always asserts supremacy of the Christ event, and in relation to righteousness he says several seemingly inconsistent things:

- He requires following the Law, but asserts that Christ is the fulfilment of the Law (Gal 2:15-21, 3:15-24, 4:1-3, Rom 9-11).
- He requires following Christ, but is neutral about the Law (Philippians 3:4-9).
- He requires following Christ but not the Law (Philippians 3:49).
- He attributes Law to Christ (Gal 3:7-11, 2:19-20).
- He asserts that Christ (grace) is necessary to follow the law (Romans 7:7-25, 2:12-25).[53]

In *Galatians,* he testifies to his own personal encounter with Christ, from whom he learned the Gospel rather than through encounter with the Apostles (1:11-18). He disparages conformity with the Law: circumcision counts for nothing with Christ (5:2); and he asserts that the whole of the law is summed up in commandment to love one another (5:15) – Christ the new creation: active faith through love (6).

In relation to the natural law, the Church usually refers to the *Romans* (2:14-16) passage. However it is not clear in the tradition that natural law is a matter of reason alone, rather it is seen as having a divine authorship. Pope Leo XIII, quoting St Thomas, appealed to the "higher reason" of the divine Lawgiver:

> But this prescription of human reason could not have the force of law unless it were the voice and the interpreter of some higher reason to which our spirit and our freedom must be subject.[54]

Indeed, the force of law consists in its authority to impose duties, to confer rights and to sanction certain behaviour: "Now all of this, clearly, could not exist in man if, as his own supreme legislator, he gave

---

[53] Troels Engber-Perdersen, *Paul and the Stoics* (Edinburgh: T&T Clark, 2000).
[54] *Libertas Praestantissimum,* n. 8.

himself the rule of his own actions."⁵⁵ And, Pope Leo concluded:

> It follows that the natural law is *itself the eternal law*, implanted in beings endowed with reason, and inclining them *towards their right action and end;* it is none other than the eternal reason of the Creator and Ruler of the universe. (St Thomas *Summa Theologiae* I-II, q. 91, a.2).⁵⁶

Pope John Paul II also connected natural law directly to divine revelation when he wrote:

> Man is able to recognize good and evil thanks to that discernment of good from evil which he himself carries out by his *reason, in particular by his reason enlightened by Divine Revelation and by faith,* through the law which God gave to the Chosen People, beginning with the commandments on Sinai. Israel was called to accept and to live out *God's law* as *a particular gift and sign of its election and of the divine Covenant,* and also as a pledge of God's blessing. Thus Moses could address the children of Israel and ask them: "What great nation is that that has a god so near to it as the Lord our God is to us, whenever we call upon him? And what great nation is there that has statutes and ordinances so righteous as all this law which I set before you this day?" (*Dt* 4:7-8).⁵⁷

Then we have the then Cardinal Ratzinger declaring that "Reason has a wax nose" and "Reason will not be saved without the faith, but the faith without reason will not be human."⁵⁸

On the other side of the coin, Pope John Paul II asserted:

> Every people has its own native and seminal wisdom which, as a true cultural treasure, tends to find voice and develop in forms which are genuinely philosophical. One example of this is the

---

⁵⁵ Ibid.
⁵⁶ Ibid.
⁵⁷ *Veritatis Splendor*, n. 44.
⁵⁸ Cardinal Joseph Ratzinger, "An address to the Congregation of the Doctrine of the Faith, 'Current Situation of Faith and Theology'" 1996, http://www.ourladyswarriors.org/dissent/ratzsitu596.htm (accessed June 18, 2008).

basic form of philosophical knowledge which is evident to this day in the postulates which inspire national and international legal systems in regulating the life of society.[59]

3.3 A Practical Partnership between Faith and Reason

In our own time, an example of that seminal wisdom is surely to be found in the International Human Rights Instruments, which:

- assert that "recognition of the inherent dignity and of the equal and inalienable rights of all members of the human family is the foundation of freedom, justice and peace in the world."
- recognise that "these rights derive from the inherent dignity of the human person."[60]

An analysis of the texts of the covenants shows that "dignity" in this context implies the inestimable worth of each member of the human family and "rights" presume to identify what is needed for human beings to flourish. The International Instruments therefore presume that human goodness is knowable and can be specified.[61]

Pope John Paul II encouraged philosophers, but again sought to connect their endeavours to Scripture:

> They should be open to the impelling questions which arise from the word of God and they should be strong enough to shape their thought and discussion in response to that challenge. Let them always strive for truth, alert to the good which truth contains. Then they will be able to formulate the genuine ethics which humanity needs so urgently at this particular time. The Church follows the

---

[59] *Fides et ratio*, n. 4.
[60] See the preambles of the "International Covenant on Civil and Political Rights"; http://www2.ohchr.org/english/law/ccpr.htm; or the "International Covenants on Economic Social and Cultural Rights"; http://www2.ohchr.org/english/law/pdf/cescr.pdf (accessed August 6, 2010).
[61] See my doctoral thesis N. Tonti-Filippini, (2000). "Human dignity: autonomy, sacredness and the international human rights instruments". PhD thesis, Department of Philosophy, The University of Melbourne, http://repository.unimelb.edu.au/10187/1396, (accessed August 6, 2010).

work of philosophers with interest and appreciation; and they should rest assured of her respect for the rightful autonomy of their discipline. I would want especially to encourage believers working in the philosophical field to illumine the range of human activity by the exercise of a reason which grows more penetrating and assured because of the support it receives from faith.[62]

The teaching of these three Popes at least, Leo XIII, John Paul II and Benedict XVI, would seem to suggest that there is to be no dichotomy between faith and reason. Rather the teaching would suggest that as philosophers we would be foolish to ignore Scripture and that our discipline should properly consider the nature of the Creator and the relationship between created and Creator, and seek to test theological propositions against reason, seeking justification rather than accepting them simply as a matter of faith. From a protestant perspective, our humanity may be too "fallen" to be able to do that, but from a Catholic perspective, we have trusted in the role of reason as an important contributor to our tradition, but not in isolation from faith and the Scriptures.

That suggests that as bioethicists, we should participate in public debate openly as Christians rather than try to engage in an exercise of pure reason. I would suggest that we should be open about our faith because subterfuge is beneath dignity and in any case, would only breed suspicion. In a pluralist society we can approach this by insisting on being willing to listen to others, willing to encourage their contribution from their own cultural beliefs, and willing to test our own Christian concepts, and in that way seek common ground by seeking to identify human goodness and the virtues. That provides a mutually respectful pathway towards seeking human transcendence together in recognition of our differences but also our commonalities.

In this respect I have been greatly encouraged by finding links between Alasdair MacIntyre and Pope John Paul II and Benedict XVI in MacIntyre's emphasis on culture and tradition and the historical

---

[62] *Fides et Ratio* n. 106.

development of ideas, and his rebuttal of the notion of pure reason building a morality from the ground up without the benefit of culture;[63] in John Paul II's recognition of native and seminal wisdom and his encouragement to philosophers to consider questions from the Word of God; and finally, in Benedict XVI's insistence on the connectedness of philosophy and theology.

A Catholic philosopher has much to contribute to Bioethics from our traditional exploration of human nature, identifying doctrines that are good for mankind and justified in human terms, and from our acceptance that we are formed by faith but willing to test propositions from revelation, knowing that God loves us and wants what is good for us.

However, I do think that a response is needed to Cardinal Ratzinger's "wax nose" concept. I would conclude that reason may not be saved without faith, but goodness is a property that is recognisable even by those who are unfamiliar with the Gospels, and that in a pluralist society we can mutually seek to identify a common understanding of human goodness.

It is relevant that in making a distinction between cardinal and theological virtues, St Thomas Aquinas claimed that all virtues other than the theological are in us by nature, according to aptitude and inchoation, but not according to perfection, and the theological virtues are from without:

> Sic ergo patet quod virtutes in nobis sunt a natura secundum aptitudinem et inchoationem, non autem secundum perfectionem: prater virtutes theologicas, quae sunt totaliter ab extrinseco.[64]

By "from without" I understand Aquinas to mean that the theological virtues are revealed to us by God rather than the product of our own reasoning.

That does raise questions about many of the issues that have been developed in *Dignitas Personae* in relation to the emphasis placed on

---

[63] Alasdair MacIntyre, *After Virtue* (Notre Dame: University of Notre Dame, 1981).
[64] St Thomae Aquinatis, *Summa Theologiae*, Prima Secundae Q. 63, Art I, English Dominican Friars Edition, 1976.

trinitarian love:

> By taking the interrelationship of these two dimensions, *the human and the divine,* as the starting point, one understands better why it is that man has unassailable value: *he possesses an eternal vocation* and *is called to share in the trinitarian love of the living God.*(n. 8)

And:

> These two dimensions of life, the natural and the supernatural, allow us to understand better the sense in which *the acts that permit a new human being to come into existence,* in which a man and a woman give themselves to each other, *are a reflection of trinitarian love.* "God, who is love and life, has inscribed in man and woman the vocation to share in a special way in his mystery of personal communion and in his work as Creator and Father" (n.9)

These passages raise something of a challenge to a natural law approach because the Trinitarian mystery is only known through Divine Revelation and these passages suggest that we should understand human love in marriage as being an imitation of the love between the divine persons and hence that the truth of that communion of persons informs our human relationships because the *imago dei* is not of single person but of a Trinity. That then suggests that we should understand human nature relationally, through the relationship of the Divine Persons, and the nuptial mystery and communio can only be fully understood through divine revelation.

This does however seem to be consistent with St Thomas's view that the theological virtues are understood only through Divine revelation.

For Catholic bioethicists, one of the most difficult aspects to argue in a pluralist context, particularly a bigoted secularist context, is the

Pauline principle[65] that underlies our morality and the related claim that there are absolute moral norms.

We generally take the Pauline Principle from the passage in *Romans* (3:8):

> Why not say – as we are being slanderously reported as saying and as some claim that we say – "Let us do evil that good may result"? Their condemnation is deserved.

From which we draw the conclusion that one must not do evil in order that good may come.

In *Veritatis Splendor* Pope John Paul II gave expression to this principle in his analysis of the moral act in terms identifying that the object of the act needs to be capable of being orientated towards God:

> Activity is morally good when it attests to and expresses the voluntary ordering of the person to his ultimate end and the conformity of a concrete action with the human good as it is acknowledged in its truth by reason. If the object of the concrete action is not in harmony with the true good of the person, the choice of that action make our will and ourselves morally evil, thus putting us in conflict with our ultimate end, the supreme good, God himself. (n.72)
>
> ... the moral life ...consists in the deliberate ordering of human acts to God, the supreme good and ultimate end (telos) of man. ... But this ordering to one's ultimate end is not something subjective, dependent solely upon one's intention. It presupposes that such acts are in themselves capable of being ordered to this end, in so far as they are in conformity with the authentic moral good of man, safeguarded by the commandments. (n.73)
>
> The morality of the human act depends primarily and fundamentally on the 'object' rationally chosen by the deliberate will ...(n. 78)

---

[65] John Finnis offers a robust defence of the Pauline Principle in his *Moral Absolutes: Tradition, Revision, and Truth* (Washington, D.C.: Catholic University of America Press, 1991).

In order to be able to grasp the object of an act which specifies that act morally, it is therefore necessary to place oneself in the perspective of the acting person. The object of the act of willing is in fact a freely chosen kind of behaviour. (n.78)

By the object of a given moral act, then, one cannot mean a process or event of the merely physical order, to be assessed on the basis of its ability to bring about a given state of affairs in the outside world. Rather that object is the proximate end of a deliberate decision which determines the act of willing on the part of the acting person. (n.78)

Expressed in these terms of a teleology that involves the Creator, it is difficult to understand the Pauline principle expressed in terms of the object of the act unless one invokes the relationship to the Creator and, in so doing, that set of beliefs about the Creator that we can only know through Divine Revelation.

I would suggest that the Pauline principle can be understood in terms of loving relationship as a desire to preserve authenticity of love. When one discusses the nature of the moral act, the notion of an absolute does emerge in the context of understanding moral acts as expressive of human love of another. Doing evil then contradicts that loving relationship but especially so when we understand love in the sense that Christ's gift of self on the Cross gave to the meaning of love.

There does seem to be a gap in natural law accounts based on reason alone when it comes to explaining absolute moral norms and the Pauline principle. This is, of course, the central issue in relation to proportionalism, situation ethics and the fundamental option (discussed later). What they lack is an adequate account of authentic human love. However it would seem that we cannot achieve an adequate account of authentic human love from reason alone. As St Thomas expresses it, the theological virtues come from without.

Basically because the moral act is to be understood in terms of communion with God, it would seem difficult to posit communion with God as our natural ultimate end, as a matter of pure reason, unless reason predicates existence of a creator who creates us for love of us (agape) and wants our love (eros) in return.[66] This notion of God seems to be peculiar to the Christian faith. It is also the case that the theological virtues (faith, hope and love), depend on both the *agapeic* and *erotic* notion of the Creator's love, and in our understanding of that love we rely on the grace of God in revealing Divine Nature to us, and we rely on Christ and his sacrifice on the Cross for our understanding of the authenticity of love as complete gift.

I am sympathetic to the task of new natural law which seeks to engage the secular world in argument based on pure reason and without assistance from revelation. It would be wonderful if with reason alone we could lead others to a position that did not contradict the moral truths of our faith. However, when it comes to the true nature of love and hence the existence of moral absolutes and the Pauline principle, I doubt that it is achievable.

From my experience in chairing government committees, I am convinced that there is a better way in which we may encourage people to seek ideal solutions to ethical problems, based on their own personal and cultural beliefs. In that respect I do not see two distinct projects in being both Christian and a philosopher. Rather, I am a Christian who is willing both to listen to others and subject my beliefs to philosophical scrutiny alongside theirs, and to ask the question, whether living according to these beliefs is a more coherent, consistent, happier and more fulfilling way to be. By this, I mean living according to the aim to give of myself to others and thus to strive to be like my Lord and Saviour.

In this respect I disagree with the double life mentality proposed by Germain Grisez, whom I nevertheless much admire, when he wrote:

> Similarly, I consider it the responsibility of the person who is both a Christian and a philosopher to remain faithful to both ways of life, to resist all demands from either side to choose between them, to deny nothing for the sake of lessening the tension, and thus to become a bridge between the gathering of

---

[66] *Deus Caritas Est,* n. 3-8.

those sons and daughters of the Church who believe and those men and women who philosophize.[67]

There should be no such division. On the other hand, I agree with Grisez when he says in the same article,

> I do not think that philosophy can begin with universal doubt. In fact, philosophers who imagine that their thinking is altogether presuppositionless have not managed to set aside all presuppositions, the better to keep them unaware of their presuppositions, the better to keep them without subjecting them to critical scrutiny.[68]

In Western culture, the greatest divide between a Catholic understanding and secularism occurs in understanding conjugality. We do need a conceptual framework to build a bridge by achieving a philosophical analysis of affectivity and communion of persons and the radical oneness of human and divine love (agape, erotic and filial), but the content for that analysis will be from Revelation.

There are different models of philosophical analysis in Western culture. Firstly there is the dominant secular view that undertakes philosophical analysis as the splintering and deconstruction of reality. In that context we can assess a philosophical work by the number of distinctions made and defended! This popular philosophical approach reduces the role of reason to narrative only. There is no objective reality and goodness is not knowable.

From a Catholic perspective what we have to offer is an alternative approach to philosophical analysis that constructively builds upon shared understanding, mutually seeking the transcendent. In that we can accept our cultures as raw data and can work to identify goodness as a common ground and knowable. That then permits us, in a culturally inclusive way, to transcend differences between religions and cultures while still founded upon those differences. That approach

---

[67] Germain Grisez, "Faith, Philosophy and Fidelity", *Fidelity*, Vol. 3, No. 8, July 1984, p. 20. In a recent email exchange Professor Grisez referred me to this article as representative of a view that he still holds.
[68] Ibid.

is especially open to the Christian notion of love, asking simply that it be considered as an alternative and asking the very practical question whether a civilisation based on a notion of love as gift of self is a better civilisation than the alternatives.

In that way we can seek to lead public reason towards accepting the propositions of *Dignitas Personae* (n .9), such as:

> Respect for that dignity is owed to every human being because each one carries in an indelible way his own dignity and value. *The origin of human life has its authentic context in marriage and in the family,* where it is generated through an act which expresses the reciprocal love between a man and a woman. Procreation which is truly responsible vis-à-vis the child to be born "must be the fruit of marriage."[69]

And that Christian marriage is rooted:

> in the natural complementarity that exists between man and woman, and is nurtured through the personal willingness of the spouses to share their entire life-project, what they have and what they are: for this reason such communion is the fruit and the sign of a profoundly human need. But in Christ the Lord, God takes up this human need, confirms it, purifies it and elevates it, leading it to perfection through the sacrament of matrimony: the Holy Spirit who is poured out in the sacramental celebration offers Christian couples the gift of a new communion of love that is the living and real image of that unique unity which makes of the Church the indivisible Mystical Body of the Lord Jesus. [70]

Thus Christian Philosophy has much to contribute to Bioethics in its exploration of human nature and in identifying doctrines that are both good for mankind and justified in human terms.

---

[69] Congregation for the Doctrine of the Faith, *Instruction Donum Vitae*, II, A, 1: *AAS* 80 (1988), 87.
[70] Ibid

3.4 Situation Ethics

Situation ethics is a view that gained some prominence in Catholic circles around the time of the Second Vatican Council and the discussion over the Papal Commission on Birth Control.

The phrase "situation ethics" is usually attributed to Joseph Fletcher, although it was used before this. Fletcher published a number of texts over a twenty-five year period.[71]

In 1952 he earned the distinction of his view being criticised by Pope Pius XII, who wrote:

> The distinctive mark of this morality is that it is in fact no way based on universal moral laws, for instance, on the Ten Commandments, but on the real and concrete conditions or circumstances in which one must act, and according to which the individual conscience has to judge and choose.[72]

Fletcher, then an Episcopalian vicar, distinguished between the old morality, which consisted of abstract principles or rules and legalistic laws or norms issued by divine or church authority or claimed as a matter of nature or essence, with his new morality which was based on experience of the context or situation in which one exercises one's conscience to give a loving response.

In his student days was Fletcher was a social activist – siding with the workers (particularly miners). He became a Christian because he saw the Church as a means of bringing social idealism to bear upon society. As he put it, "It was not Christianity which led me to my social ideals; ... my social ideals led me to Christianity."

---

[71] *Morals and Medicine* (N.J.: Princeton University Press, 1954); *Situation Ethics: The New Morality*, (Philadelphia: Westminster Press, 1966); *Moral Responsibility: Situation Ethics at Work*, (Philadelphia: Westminster Press, 1967); *The Situation Ethics Debate*, with Harvey Cox, (Philadelphia: Westminster Press, 1968); *Hello Lovers: An Introduction to Situation Ethics*, with Thomas A. Wassmer SJ, (New York: Corpus Books,1970); *Situation Ethics: True or False*, with John Montgomery, (Minneapolis: Dimension Books, 1972); *The Ethics of Genetic Control: Ending Reproductive Roulette*, (New York: Doubleday, 1974).

[72] Pius XII, Allocution on "New Morality," April 19, 1952, *Acta Apostolica Sedis* Volume 44, 1952, p. 270.

Most of his writings and activities during the time of his ministry were to do with his social theology. He came to realise that he did not believe in doctrinaire solutions:

"At bottom I was still convinced by the case for pragmatism, in both the cognitive and ethical sense, which I had long since accepted as a convinced pupil of James and Dewey."

His rejection of the doctrinaire and the dogmatic bore its fruit in his best-seller, *Situation Ethics*. As he explains, its thesis was set within the context of Christian rhetoric, but situation ethics as a theory of moral action is utterly independent of Christian presuppositions or beliefs.[73]

By 1970 Fletcher had settled firmly for the consequentialist position that the right thing to do in any case is whatever will maximize human benefit, regardless of supposedly relevant but abstract moral rules. He thus rejects a systematic Christian ethics. The context or situation is all important and cannot be anticipated completely in any systematic ethics. He thus described systematic orthodoxy as legalism. At the same time, Fletcher declared himself against antinomianism – holding no principles at all. Instead, situationism confronts a situation "armed" with principles/maxims from one's community, but ready to compromise "if love seems better served by doing so."[74]

He argued that the person and his or her situation is unique and the only categorical commandment is to love. Some of his sayings were:

- Love Only is Always Good.
- Love is the only Norm.
- Love and Justice are the same.
- Love is not Liking.
- Love justifies the Means.
- Love Decides There and Then.
- "Love" is not sentimental love, but an act of the will – willing the well-being of the other(s).

---

[73] Joseph Fletcher, *Situation Ethics: The New Morality* (Philadelphia: Westminster Press, 1966) p. 82.
[74] Ibid., p. 26.

- Value is relative to persons and persons are relative to society.
- Conscience is a verb not a noun.
- The ultimate criterion is "agapeic love."[75]

In answer to the question, "How do we know the loving thing to do?" Fletcher suggested that "Our situation ethics frankly joins forces with Mill ... We choose what is most 'useful' for the most people."[76] He argued that the rule of thumb for loving is "seek the best welfare and deepest happiness of the most people in the situation."[77]

In response to the question, "What is distinctive about 'Christian' ethics?" Fletcher argued that the Christ Factor and his complete gift of himself on the Cross makes our understanding of love different. Later however he abandoned this and declared himself a humanist: "Whatever helps people is good, whatever hurts them is evil." He contrasted this with theism: "Whatever does the will of God is good, what ignores or flouts God is evil." Fletcher thought that there is a possible way out for theism if it acknowledges that God wills man's good, but he asserts that most Christians condemn this kind of ethics.[78]

There are a number of problems with Situation Ethics. First, it sets up a false description of Christianity in criticising the latter. Consideration of the context has always been part of the tradition, which is not solely rule-based. The principle of double effect, in particular, allows an assessment to be made of the consequences, and the intended and foreseen consequence should be assessed as part of determining the rightness or otherwise of an individual act in order to understand the act involved and the possible "sinfulness" of an individual in performing it. Casuistry has also been part of the tradition in which we are to treat like cases alike. The major difference is that

---

[75] Ibid.
[76] Ibid., p. 115.
[77] Joseph Fletcher, *The Situation Ethics Debate*, with Harvey Cox, (Philadelphia: Westminster Press, 1968) p. 260.
[78] Joseph Fletcher "Ethics and Euthanasia" in *Regulating How We Die: The Ethical, Medical and Legal Issues Surrounding Physician-Assisted Suicide*, Linda L. Emanuel, ed. Cambridge, MA: Harvard University Press, 1998.

Situation Ethics regards each case as unique, so that general principles do not hold.

In Fletcher's account of Situation Ethics, the notion of love seems devoid of content. The predicted consequences are not the only factor to be considered in relation to whether an act is an act of love. As any spouse can attest, the meaning given to an act by the parties to it is crucial. Fletcher attaches no weight to what I referred to earlier as the intransitive effects of an act. My acts express who I am and when I do evil that determines who I am. Finally, because he embraces utilitarianism, Fletcher's account is open to all the criticisms against utilitarianism provided earlier, including the difficulty of aggregating people for the purpose of evaluating consequences and accepting the resultant injustices.

3.5 Proportionalism and Double-Effect Reasoning

Double-effect reasoning, particularly as it appears in St. Thomas Aquinas,[79] is usually given as the source of the perspective of moral theology known as "proportionalism." A key proponent of proportionalism has been Joseph Fuchs,[80] who argued that there are objective norms, but they are culturally and historically conditioned, not universal. Further, he argued that all moral norms must admit of exceptions, and he adopted the term "pre-moral" evil to describe evil defined by a moral norm prior to assessing the overall good and evil aspects of an act. On this view, it is only when that balance has been achieved that one can determine whether an act is reasonable or not. He wrote:

> What must be determined is the significance of the action as value or non-value for the individual, for interpersonal

---

[79] St Thomas Aquinas, *Summa Theologiae* II-II, q. 64, a. 7.
[80] Joseph Fuchs, "The Absoluteness of Behavioural Moral Norms" *Gregorianum*, 1971 cf. Zachary C Eyster, *Imagining ethics: re-imagining salvation: Josef Fuchs, fundamental option, and the soteriological implications thereof* Villanova University, 2009.

relations and for human society, in connection ... with the total reality of man and his society and in view of his whole culture. Furthermore the priority and urgency of different values implied must be weighed.

This view differs from Situation Ethics[81] in that it takes into account the meaning of an act and thus accepts that there may be intrinsic evil in an act. It differs also, however, from a traditional Christian or biblical view, which holds that some acts, such as direct killing of the innocent, are always wrong. In Fuchs' view, such evil is "premoral" and is to be balanced with the good and evil consequences in a given situation.

A number of theologians have taken a similar view, including Jack Mahoney SJ, Charles Curran and Richard McCormick.

McCormick has made a significant contribution to discussion of Bioethics. I met him at his home in Washington in 1984 at the time that in vitro fertilization had recently been widely accepted as a remedy for infertility and the morality of the procedure was under intense discussion. I suggested that the technology involved enormous loss of nascent human life including deliberate destruction of embryos selected for unwanted characteristics or because growth appeared too slow or too fast to be normal. I also suggested that inherently the technology involved a relationship of domination between the technologist and the embryo in which the embryo was a product of a making, and subject to quality control. I argued that the equality that is present when a child originates from an act of love as an equal third party and an embodiment of that love was missing in the case of the laboratory generation of life.[82]

McCormick responded by saying that such concerns were a matter of caution, but had to be weighed against the desire for the couple to have a child and the great good of the coming to be of a new life. This

---

[81] Joseph Fletcher, *Moral Responsibility: Situation Ethics at Work* (Philadelphia: Westminster Press, 1967).
[82] Nicholas Tonti-Filippini, *Ethics and the Treatment of Infertility* (Melbourne: Holy Name Press, 1983); Nicholas Tonti-Filippini "IVF: the role of the technician" in *Persona Verita e Morale*, (Rome: Citta Nuova Editrice 1986).

view was implicit in his essay "Ambiguity in Moral Choice," in his edited collection *Doing Evil to Achieve Good*,[83] and it was argued later in *How Brave a New World? Dilemmas in Bioethics*.[84]

McCormick has published extensively in moral theology and bioethics but there does not appear to be any systematic presentation of his theory. Proportionalism, as a view, seemed to arise around the time of the Papal Commission on Birth Control. The majority report argued that to take another's life is a sin not because life is under the exclusive dominion of God, but because it is contrary to right reason *unless there is a question of a good of a higher order*; it is licit to sacrifice a life for the good of the community.[85]

This argument was attributed to St Thomas Aquinas who taught that one could take the life of another in self defence:

> Therefore this act, since one's intention is to save one's own life, is not unlawful, seeing that it is natural to everything to keep itself in "being," as far as possible. And yet, though proceeding from a good intention, an act may be rendered unlawful, if it be out of proportion to the end.[86]

The standard rendition of this principle is roughly as follows:

1. The act itself must be morally good or at least indifferent.
2. The agent may not positively will the bad effect but may permit it. If he could attain the good effect without the bad effect he should do so. The bad effect is sometimes said to be indirectly voluntary.
3. The good effect must flow from the action at least as immediately (in the order of causality, though not necessarily in the order of time) as the bad effect. In other

---

[83] Richard McCormick and Paul Ramsey, *Doing Evil to Achieve Good: Moral Choice in Conflict Situations* (Chicago: Loyola University Press, 1978, pp.7-53.
[84] Richard McCormick, *How Brave a New World? Dilemmas in Bioethics* (New York: Doubleday, 1985).
[85] "The Question is not Closed," in *The Birth-Control Debate*, ed. Robert Hoyt (Kansas City, MO: The National Catholic Reporter, 1969), p. 69.
[86] St Thomas Aquinas, *Summa Theologiae*, II-II, q. 64, a. 7.

words, the good effect must be produced directly by the action, not by the bad effect. Otherwise the agent would be using a bad means to a good end, which is never allowed.
4. The good effect must be sufficiently desirable to compensate for the allowing of the bad effect.

Most recently McCormick wrote:

> When contemporary theologians say that certain values or disvalues in our actions can be justified by a proportionate reason, they are not saying that morally wrong actions (ex objecto) can be justified by their end. They are saying that an act cannot be classified morally simply by looking at its *material circa quam*, or at its object in a very narrow and restricted sense. This is precisely what tradition has done in the categories exempted from teleological assessment (e.g. contraception and sterilization). It does this in no other area. I further argued that the term "object" was so inconsistently used sometimes needed to decide what should count to fit those categories. Actions that when abstractly considered, contain some important deformity or disorder but are made morally right by the circumstances, e.g, in St Thomas's words, "The killing and the beating of a man involve some deformity in their object." But if it added to this that an evildoer is killed for the sake of justice or that a delinquent is beaten for punishment then the action is not a sin, rather it is virtuous.[87]

As authority for this passage, McCormick cites *Quaestiones Quodlibetales*.[88] However, as William E May has pointed out,[89] Aquinas immediately goes on to say in this passage that there are some kinds of human acts that "have deformity inseparably annexed to them, such

---

[87] Richard McCormick, "Classification Through Dialogue" in Richard McCormick and Charles Curran *The Historical Development of Moral Theology in the United States* (New Jersey: Paulist Press, 1999), pp. 193-4.
[88] St Thomas Aquinas, *Quaestiones Quodlibetales*, 9, q. 7, a. 2.
[89] William E. May, "Moral Theologians and Veritatis Splendor", http://www.ewtn.com/library/THEOLOGY/MORALVS.HTM, (accessed August 6, 2010).

as fornication, adultery, and others of this sort."[90] Aquinas explicitly affirms that some actions, as specified by their objects, are intrinsically evil, and corresponding to them are absolute moral norms.[91]

Biblically, it is clear that the Decalogue provides a set of exceptionless norms and far from weakening them, Jesus in the Sermon on the Mount explains them in terms that are, if anything, more demanding, such as adultery in the heart and, with respect to the fifth commandment, anger. He prefaces his comments by saying:

> Do not think that I have come to abolish the Law or the Prophets; I have not come to abolish them but to fulfill them. I tell you the truth, until heaven and earth disappear, not the smallest letter, not the least stroke of a pen, will by any means disappear from the Law until everything is accomplished. Anyone who breaks one of the least of these commandments and teaches others to do the same will be called least in the kingdom of heaven, but whoever practices and teaches these commands will be called great in the kingdom of heaven. For I tell you that unless your righteousness surpasses that of the Pharisees and the teachers of the law, you will certainly not enter the kingdom of heaven. (Matthew 6:17-20)

Double-effect reasoning may be understood by distinguishing between the following hypothetical examples attributed to Philippa Foot.[92]

A trolley is running out of control down a track. In its path are five people who have been tied to the track by an evil philosopher. Fortunately, you can flip a switch, which will lead the trolley down a different track to safety. Unfortunately, there is a single person tied

---

[90] "Quaedam enim sunt quae habent deformitatem inseparabiliter annexam, ut fornicatio, adulterium, et aliae huiusmodi, quae nullo modo bene fieri possunt." St Thomas Aquinas, *Quaestiones Quodlibetales*, 9, q. 7, a. 2.
[91] Ibid.
[92] Philippa Foot, *The Problem of Abortion and the Doctrine of the Double Effect* in *Virtues and Vices* (Oxford: Basil Blackwell, 1978).

to that track. Most people will accept that you can and should flip the switch as the only way of saving life even though by doing so you permit or indirectly cause the death of the one person in order to save the five. But this is not just a utilitarian calculation of taking one life to save five. What makes the option acceptable to many of us is that the one person who dies does so as an indirect effect of an act the purpose of which is to save life. The direct object of the act is to save life, the act is still an act of killing, but the killing of the one is indirect. It is not the means and it is not the purpose of the act.

Foot also describes a case in which a group of rioters are demanding that a culprit be found for a certain crime and they are threatening to kill five hostages if the culprit is not found. The real culprit being unknown, the judge sees himself as able to prevent the death of the five by framing one innocent person and having him executed. Most of us would not find framing the innocent man to be an acceptable choice despite the fact that four lives are saved. This case is the same as the trolley case in terms of consequences, the lives lost and saved, but it differs in that the death is intended as a means and is not merely permitted. The act by the judge is a direct killing rather than indirect because it is a means to the end. In the case of the trolley, the death of the one man is indirect and merely permitted or merely foreseen as a result of diverting the trolley to save the lives of the five.

McCormick accepts that these two cases are different, and that the direct and indirect distinction is important. He argues that the moral guilt of the mob in being willing to take the five lives unjustly is not altered by the decision of the judge. His decision, however, does lessen the moral disvalue of their action because it does reduce the loss of life. But our concern about the morality of the judge's decision remains. We are appalled, McCormick says, because taking a life in these circumstances would encourage similar acts of injustice and thus render more lives vulnerable. If the direct killing were rendered permissible by balancing the consequences, then this would encourage or foster similar injustices and that would be a long-term disaster. So on that score, direct killing should be excluded because there would be worse long-term consequences if we did not uphold the difference between deliberate and incidental killing or direct and indirect killing.[93]

On that basis, McCormick concludes that the teleological character of all our norms does not eliminate the relevance of the distinction between direct and indirect where non-moral values and disvalues are involved. The relationship of the evil that occurs to my will or purpose says a great deal about the meaning of my action, its repercussions and implications, and therefore whether the action is in the long term good.[94]

On this analysis, the judge's act is wrong because it is a direct killing, but the direct killing is wrong because if direct killings were considered permissible, then this would have many other consequences tolerating other acts of direct killing and thus making lives much more vulnerable. In other words, the evil of direct killing is not in the directness of the killing but in the consequences that would result from the belief that direct killing is not wrong.

Judith Jarvis Thomson[95] proposes a variation of the trolley story:

> As before, a trolley is hurtling down a track towards five people. You are on a bridge under which it will pass, and you can stop it by dropping a heavy weight in front of it. As it happens, there is a very fat man next to you – your only way to stop the trolley is to push him over the bridge and onto the track, killing him to save five.

Many would put this account in the same category as the story of the judge framing the innocent man. Many would hold that the death is a means to the end and therefore cannot be considered to be indirect because it is necessary to attain the desired result. One certainly cannot

---

[93] Richard McCormick, "Ambiguity in Moral Choice" in Richard McCormick and Paul Ramsey *Doing Evil to Achieve Good: Moral Choice in Conflict Situations* (Chicago: Loyola University, 1978) p. 33.
[94] Ibid.
[95] Judith Jarvis Thomson, "Killing, Letting Die, and the Trolley Problem", *The Monist*, Vol. 59, 1976, pp. 204-17.

describe pushing the man over the bridge as merely permitting his death. So then, it may be asked, would it make a difference if the fat man was in fact the evil philosopher who had placed the five in danger and released the trolley in the first place? What if the philosopher is not in fact evil but simply mentally deranged and has no sense of the wrong of what he has done?

The distinction that St Thomas Aquinas makes is between two effects of the one act, saving one's life and slaying an aggressor by the use of violence against him. What makes the slaying indirect is that the act of the will is self defence, not that the act is not an act against the aggressor. There is no doubt that St Thomas meant an act of violence against the aggressor:

> Now moral acts take their species according to what is intended, and not according to what is beside the intention, since this is accidental as explained above... Accordingly the act of self defence may have two effects, one is the saving of one's life, the other is the slaying of the aggressor. Therefore this act, since one's intention is to save one's life, is not unlawful, seeing that it is natural to everything to keep itself in being, as far as possible.[96]

He goes on to make a point about proportionality and it is this point that is the focus of the proportionalists:

> And yet through proceeding from a good intention, an act may be rendered unlawful, if it be out of proportion to the end. Wherefore if a man, in self defense uses more than necessary violence, it will be unlawful: whereas if he repel force with moderation his defense will be lawful, because according to the jurists, it is lawful to repel force by force, provided one does not

---

[96] "Morales autem actus recipient speciem secundum Id quod est praeter intentionem, cum sit per accidens, ut ex supradictus patet. Ex actu igitur alicuius seipsum defendentis duplex effectus sequi potest; unus quidem conservatio propriae vitae; alius autem occisio inadventis. Actus igitur huiusmodi ex hoc quod intenditur conservatio propriae vitae, non habet rationem illicit: cum hoc sit cuilibet natural quod se conservet in esse quantum potest." St Thomas Aquinas *Summa Theologica* II II Q. 64, Art. 7.

exceed the limits of a blameless defense.[97]

For Aquinas this issue of proportionality only follows if the nature of the act itself is not evil. Pope John Paul II teaches that that which is directly willed must be capable of being oriented towards God[98]. One must also consider whether the consequences of what one does are just and whether the evil effects are not out of proportion to the good that one intends. However whatever about the consequences, an act will be considered evil if what is directly willed is evil.

Evangelium Vitae also refers to St Alphonsus in relation to killing in self defence, although in my close reading of St Alphonsus' text *Theologia Moralis*, l. III, tr. 4, c. 1, dub.3., I cannot find the passage that *EV* refers to (it is, admittedly, a rather long passage and my Latin is rusty). However I did find in his *Homo Apostolicus Tr 1, No. 1* where he makes the point that a human act is to be judged good or bad according to an understanding of the good as it is pursued by the will, and not according to the material object of the act.

The distinction that the Magisterium has engaged is based on determining what is the immediate object, the means or the direct intention. In the language of *Veritatis Splendor*, the issue is what is the immediate object of the act and whether it is capable of being oriented towards God[99]. In the case of killing in self defence, this is a distinction between what is directly willed in an act, and the fact that the act also kills someone. Because the direct object is to save life, that the aggressor dies as a result of the act is considered to be permissible. It is important to acknowledge that double-effect reasoning does not allow one to will the evil directly.

Imagine that I could save many lives by spending an inheritance on them, but in fact standing between the saving of those lives and the

---

[97] "Potest tamen aliquius actus ex bona intentione proveniens illicitus reddi si non sit proportionatus fini. Et ideo si aliquis ad defendendum propriam vitam utatur maiori violentia quam opoteat, erit illicitum. Si vero moderate violentiam repellat, erit licita defebsio: nam secundum iura, vim vi repellere licet cum moderamine inculpate tutelage." Ibid.
[98] *Veritatis Splendor*, n. 78.
[99] Ibid.

inheritance is the fact that an older brother is due to inherit the money and intends to use it sustaining his profligate life style. Killing him so that the money goes to saving lives could not be considered an act in defence of those lives because it is an act of killing, The death is a means to a good end, but the direct object of the act is not saving life but killing him. The good intended consequences do not make the evil act permissible.

As Pope John Paul II expresses it:

> The reason why a good intention is not itself sufficient, but a correct choice of actions is also needed, is that the human act depends on its object, whether that object is *capable or not of being ordered* to God, to the One who "alone is good," and thus brings about the perfection of the person. An act is therefore good if its object is in conformity with the good of the person with respect for the goods morally relevant for him.[100]

St Thomas observes that "it often happens that man acts with a good intention, but without spiritual gain, because he lacks a good will. Let us say that someone robs in order to feed the poor: in this case, even though the intention is good, the uprightness of the will is lacking. Consequently, no evil done with a good intention can be excused. 'There are those who say: And why not do evil that good may come? Their condemnation is just' (*Rom* 3:8)."[101]

Contemporary proportionalism seems to have its origins in the history of the issue of contraception and the Papal Commission on Birth Control[102] which preceded the papal encyclical *Humanae Vitae* in 1968. Dissent from the teaching on contraception since tends to have adopted proportionalism. Peter Knauer is often quoted as the source of proportionalism. According to Knauer, "some acts which would have

---

[100] Ibid.
[101] St Thomas Aquinas, *In Duo Praecepta Caritatis et in Decem Legis Praecepta. De Dilectione Dei: Opuscula Theologica*, II, No. 1168, (Ed. Taurinen,1954), 250. cf *Veritatis Splendor*, n. 78.
[102] Papal Commission on Birth Control, *The Tablet*, April 22, 1967, pp. 449-454; April 29, 1967, pp. 478-485; May 6, 1967, pp. 510-513; September 21, 1968, pp. 949-951.

to be judged morally wrong according to the traditional prohibition against intending evil, ought instead to be judged morally licit so long as the good pursued is commensurate to the evil purposefully caused."[103] His principal thesis was that moral evil consisted in doing physical evil without commensurate reason. He argued, on the basis of the above passage from St Thomas on self-defence, that what made the physical act of killing someone in self-defence permissible was the presence of a commensurate reason – in this case the saving of life. He argued that the meaning of that act was therefore not derived from its external effect – killing the aggressor, but really that aspect of the act that is willed – the saving of life. The saving of the life is a commensurate reason that changes the meaning of an act which would otherwise simply be a slaying.

The following are examples from the literature that clarify what is meant by double-effect reasoning.

> a) A surgeon operates to remove an aggressive tumour on a woman's face and in the process leaves her with a mutilating injury to her face. Most of us would accept that what he did is properly described as life saving and that the damage that he has done to her face is a side effect and not something directly willed even though he would reasonably have predicted that that would be the consequence of the incision that he made to remove the tissue. This is a legitimate application of double-effect reasoning. The act can be described as causing a mutilation to the woman's face. The mutilation is a direct physical result of the act. But this is not the description that is most apt for moral purposes. The immediate object is to remove the cancerous tissue that would threaten the woman's life.
>
> b) As the Russian armies drove westward to meet the Americans and British at the Elbe, a Soviet patrol picked up a Mrs. Bergmeier foraging food for her three children. Unable even to get word to

---

[103] Peter Knauer, "The Hermeneutic Function of the Double Effect Reasoning," first published in French in 1965 and in English in the journal *Natural Law Forum,* Vol 12, 1967, pp. 132-62.

the children, she was taken off to a POW camp in Ukraine. Her husband had been captured in the Battle of the Bulge and taken to a POW camp in Wales. When he was returned to Berlin, he spent months rounding up his children, although they couldn't find their mother. She more than anything else was needed to reknit them as a family in that dire situation of hunger, chaos and fear. Meanwhile, in Ukraine, Mrs. Bergmeier learned through a sympathetic commandant that her husband and family were trying to keep together and find her. But the rules allowed them to release her to Germany only if she was pregnant, in which case she would be returned as a liability. She turned things over in her mind and finally asked a friendly Volga German camp guard to impregnate her, which he did. Her condition being medically verified, she was sent back to Berlin and to her family. They welcomed her with open arms, even when she told them how she had managed it. And when the child was born, they all loved him because of what they had done for them. After the christening, they met up with their local pastor and discussed the morality of the situation.[104]

Most moralists do not consider this to be an example of double-effect reasoning because the good effect happens only as a result of the bad effect. In other words, the act of adultery is the *means* to the good end of reuniting the family. For double-effect reasoning to apply, the good effect must not be dependant on the bad effect. In other words, the end cannot justify the means.

What makes St Thomas' account of self-defence acceptable is that the use of violence is to save life, the aim being to stop the aggressor. That the act of violence also kills the aggressor is a result of stopping the aggressor rather than being directly willed. Obviously there is a fine line between killing the aggressor in order to stop him and stopping the aggressor and in the process causing his death. On a traditional interpretation of the principle, the first would not be permissible but the

---

[104] Joseph Fletcher, *Situation Ethics: The New Morality* (Philadelphia, PA: Westminster Press, 1966) p. 1.

second may be, provided that there is no less drastic way of stopping the aggressor that would not have killed him – the proportionality or justice criterion requiring moderation.

The point that a proportionalist is likely to make is that the same physical, bodily reality of killing may be several different intersubjective realities: murder, waging war, administering the death penalty, self-defence, suppressing an insurrection or saving the life of a mother with an ectopic pregnancy. Taking something from another may intersubjectively be stealing, borrowing, satisfying dire need, repossessing one's property.[105]

In this view, we may not classify an act as evil until we have explored its intersubjectivity. The physical act is not right or wrong of itself until we understand its intersubjective context. Proportionalists classify the evil done by an act prior to an assessment of its intersubjectivity as "premoral evil." They argue that we cannot judge the moral nature of an act on the basis of the physical act alone.

By contrast, a position that classifies some moral norms as absolute, such as the commandments of the Decalogue, does not describe them as mere physical acts. When it came to expressing the fifth commandment in *Evangelium Vitae*, Pope John Paul II expressed the norm in the following way:

> Therefore, by the authority which Christ conferred upon Peter and his Successors, and in communion with the Bishops of the Catholic Church, I confirm that the direct and voluntary killing of an innocent human being is always gravely immoral. This doctrine, based upon that unwritten law which man, in the light of reason, finds in his own heart (cf. Rom 2:14-15), is reaffirmed by Sacred Scripture, transmitted by the Tradition of the Church and taught by the ordinary and universal Magisterium.[106]

---

[105] Richard McCormick and Paul Ramsey, *Doing Evil to Achieve Good: Moral Choice in Conflict Situations,* (Chicago: Loyola University, 1978) pp.7-53.
[106] *Evangelium Vitae,* n. 57.

"Direct and voluntary killing" is not a description of a physical act alone but qualifies the intentionality or object of the act.

There is some truth in what is claimed by proportionalists. The mere physical description of an act does not provide sufficient information for moral assessment. We do need to know the mind of the acting person.

Peter Knauer offers the complex notion of what he calls "commensurate reason". For him it is not just a matter of any countervailing reason of significant gravity being enough to justify the physical evil done. He insists that the value being realised by measures involving physical evil must not be undermined or contradicted by that evil. Thus for an act to be immoral because it is contraceptive, it must be shown that the act in the last analysis does not serve the end of preservation and deepening of marital love, but in the long term subverts it. The refusal to bear a child in that instance is only commensurately grounded if it is ultimately in the interests of the otherwise possible children.[107]

Some claim that proportionalism is mistaken because the premoral evil and the commensurate reason are incommensurable. Knauer's account of commensurability, however, is not open to this claim. He requires the reason and the evil to be connected to the same goods. Thus Knauer appears to interpret double-effect reasoning to contain the notion that one may not directly will *moral* evil in order to achieve good and what constitutes *moral* evil would be a physical evil for which there was no commensurate good effect on the same goods that define that physical evil.

Thus one could contraceive by acting against the possibility of bearing a child if the good of bearing children was also served by not having a child at this time, or if suppressing the unitive dimension of love expressed in having a child who embodies that love and whose coming to be gives witness to the fruitfulness of divine love was outweighed by the fact that the suppression facilitated a deepening of that unitive love by, for instance, permitting the couple more time to

---

[107] Knaeur, op. cit., cf. McCormick.

express that love for each other and attain greater fruitfulness.

The idea is that these consequences alter the nature of the evil involved so that in fact what is directly chosen is not, on balance, destructive of the goods that would otherwise define the evil. This would therefore not be a turning against a good but in fact a pursuit of it. What makes the fatal act of self defence permissible is that the act is done to preserve life, and this changes the meaning of the physical event of the aggressor's death.

Thus this argument may not be open to the claim that Grisez[108] and others have made that proportionalism allows us to turn directly against the good. For Knaeur, the physical evil of acting against a good may be justified by acting in service of the same good. Grisez claims in response that Knauer has had to separate moral intent from psychological intent. McCormick admits that that is so and that it makes it difficult for Knauer to deal with cases like the Mrs. Berhmeier case given above. The good at stake in her adultery is the love between her and her husband, and the unity of their relationship, but the benefits of her act are intended to serve exactly that good and to bring them back together. There would therefore appear to be a commensurate reason involving the same goods that would make the physical evil of the adultery not a moral evil: any damage to their love from the adultery is overcome by the act being a service towards permitting them to come together again.

What this latter case illustrates is that the Knauer version of the double effect reasoning seemingly makes the direct and indirect distinction redundant. The end can in fact justify the means provided the same goods are at issue.

On this account, one could directly take life to save life, but one could not directly take life for any other reason. Direct abortion to save the life of a mother for whom continued pregnancy was a life risk, such as during the treatment for acute Leukaemia, when miscarriage would be likely to occur when her blood platelets were lowest and thus

---

[108] Germain Grisez et al, *Abortion: The Myths, the Realities and the Arguments*, Washington: Corpus Books, 1970, p. 331.

fatal haemorrhage would be likely, would in that case be permissible because the same good, the good of life, is at stake.

The problem for many moralists in this case is that direct abortion remains a direct killing, an offence against the fifth commandment, and what Pope John Paul II defined as the direct and voluntary killing of an innocent human being.[109]

McCormick's initial response to Knauer was critical. He saw that Knauer made the direct/indirect distinction redundant, and did away with the concept of the "object of the act" as it had been understood psychologically, replacing it with a moral notion that treated the good at stake as a single item so that the overall effect on that good could override the evil effect with respect to that same good. Later however McCormick seems to have come to a position in which he is prepared to accept these difficulties with Knauer's position.

McCormick recognised the incommensurability of basic goods and therefore the impossibility of identifying a simple maximisation of good and minimising of evil, but Knauer's approach would seem to have avoided that difficulty by the way in which commensurate reason is defined so that the good and the evil effects relate to the same good. Thus the theory limits the application to conflict cases such that a value of the same kind and at least equal to that sacrificed is at stake, and there is no less harmful way of protecting the value here and now.

In McCormick's most recent account, evil is permissible if there is a proportionate reason for which the good sought will not be undermined by the proposed action; that is, if there is a proportionate reason that will not be undermined if the means chosen involve evil effects that involve that same good. He refers to an "association of, or necessary connection between the goods" to help to explain how one good might be undermined through harm to another.[110]

---

[109] *Evangelium Vitae*, n. 73.
[110] Richard McCormick, "A Commentary on the Commentaries" in *Doing Evil*, op. cit., p. 238.

McCormick returns to the Mrs Bergmeier case.[111] He says that there is an absence of a proportionate reason for her adultery because there is an absence of a connectedness between the sexual intimacy of her adultery with the good she seeks as a result of it, her freedom. He argues similarly the immorality of obliteration bombing such as Nagasaki and Hiroshima because,

> Making innocent (noncombatant) persons the object of our targeting is a form of extortion in international affairs that contains an implicit denial of human freedom. Human freedom is undermined when extortionary actions are accepted and elevated and universalized. Because such freedom is an associated good upon which the very good of life heavily depends, undermining it in the manner of my defense of life is undermining life itself – is disproportionate.[112]

The point seems to be both that there is an absence of a connection between the goods that would permit one to be a commensurate or proportionate reason for permitting the other, and that permitting direct killing produces greater long-term harm for human freedom and life.

The distinction between direct and indirect thus retains its significance in that killing with a proportionate reason for doing so can be considered to be indirect, as the act is directly in service of the good that is affected by the evil indirect consequence; and that permitting direct killing without a proportionate reason will in the long term result in greater harm.

Later, however, McCormick comes to reject the distinction between direct and indirect intention altogether. McCormick refers to sterility caused to remove a cancerous uterus as a life-saving procedure and sterility caused in order to control conception as a marriage-stabilizing and family stabilizing procedure. The former is an example often given to illustrate indirect intention and is usually held to be permissible even though sterility is the result. The immediate object is to save life. The second example is usually considered to be direct and

---
[111] Ibid.
[112] Ibid., p. 236.

impermissible because sterilization is a means to the end. However of these two cases McCormick writes, "Whether either intervention is justified depends not on the directness or indirectness of intentionality, but on the goodness of the end and the proportion between the means chosen and the end."[113]

There are a variety of problems for proportionalism including:

- How far into the future do you consider consequences?
- Who counts in considering consequences?
- How do you evaluate different consequences against each other?
- How do you explain free choice?[114]

McCormick is not prepared to give the direct-indirect distinction away completely and writes in favour of it: "... even though our spontaneous and instinctive moral judgments can be affected by cultural distortions and can be confused with rather obvious but deeply ingrained conventional fears and biases, still they remain a more reliable test of the humanizing and dehumanizing, of the morally right and wrong, of proportion, than our discursive arguments."[115]

There is currently further, not completely unrelated tension over double-effect reasoning and the concept of direct killing. Germain Grisez has claimed that craniotomy in the circumstances of arrested labour is not direct killing.

> In times past complications of delivery raised serious problems. Now where medical facilities are available such difficulties are rare, most difficult cases are prevented by timely surgery. However, if it were impossible to prevent the mother's death (or, worse, the death of both) except by cutting up and removing the child piecemeal, it seems to me that this death-dealing deed

---

[113] Ibid., p. 241.
[114] I am indebted to Ray Campbell for these points which were made in a lecture that he gave to my graduate students at the John Paul II institute for Marriage and Family in Melbourne, Summer 2007.
[115] Richard McCormick, "A Commentary on the Commentaries" in *Doing Evil*, op. cit., p. 251.

could be done without the killing itself coming within the scope of the intention. The very deed which deals death also (by hypothesis) initiates a unified and humanly indivisible physical human process which saves life.[116]

Originally Grisez's argument appears to have been based on an action theory that analyses an act as being an indivisible set of constituent parts.[117] In this case, according to Grisez, the surgeon performing craniotomy performs just one human act to save the life of the mother, but that act has a number of identifiable physical acts. He argued that it is only the human act, saving the life of the mother, that is subject to scrutiny. This chosen human act has an end, an intended end, namely, the preservation of the mother's life. The individual physical acts are not human acts and therefore do not fall under the scope of the intention. Therefore the act of dismembering the foetus is not a human act, rather it is part of the indivisible series of physical acts of saving the life of the mother. He held that it is therefore not a direct killing, because the death of the child is not required in order to save the life.[118]

On revisiting the issue, however, Finnis, Grisez and Boyle[119] appear to have repudiated that approach, but without changing their view about craniotomy. They say that the concept of indivisibility has not been used since 1970 and that it was a false step caused by the failure to appreciate the decisive significance of the perspective of the acting person.[120]

Grisez is a strong critic of proportionalism, but one could be forgiven for wondering how his original account of the indivisibility of the moral act essentially differs from McCormick's claim that "an

---

[116] Germain Grisez, *Abortion: The Myths, the Realities, and the Arguments*, (New York: Corpus Books, 1970), p. 370.
[117] Jean Porter, "'Direct' and 'Indirect' in Grisez's Moral Theory", *Theological Studies*, Vol 57, 1996, p. 612.
[118] Grisez, op. cit., pp. 333, 340, 341.
[119] John M. Finnis, Germain G. Grisez, & Joseph M. Boyle, "'Direct' and 'Indirect': A Reply to Critics of Our Action Theory", *Thomist*, Vol 65, No. 1, 2001, pp. 1-44.
[120] Ibid.

act cannot be classified morally simply by looking at its *material circa quam,* or at its object in a very narrow and restricted sense," and we must look at the intersubjectivity of the act in order to determine whether it is a moral evil. More to the point, why is Grisez's current analysis of the subjectivity of the human act not open to the same criticism that he made of proportionalists: that it involves separating moral intent from psychological intent?

A concern I have with the Finnis, Boyle and Grisez analysis of the account of the moral act in *Veritatis Splendor* is that they seem to interpret the document in a way that suits their own argument, in particular the passage:

> By the object of a given moral act, one cannot mean a process or an event of the merely physical order, to be assessed on its ability to bring about a given state of affairs in the world.[121]

They say of this passage, referring to St Thomas, that the species of the moral act as good or bad is not in its species *in genere naturae* but in its species *in genere moris*. They argue that it is necessary to get beyond common-sense accounts of what is being done and factors such as causal sequences, to which they give an unreflective priority over the perspective of the acting person.[122]

However, they seem to deny any role at all for the physical reality in determining the psychological reality. The issue is certainly to assess the act from the perspective of the acting person, but the latter cannot be completely unrelated to the reality of what he or she does. My concern is that in claiming that the narrowing of the child's head is the immediate object in order to save the life of the mother, the description omits a large part of what would be in the mind of the surgeon. "Narrowing the baby's head" is only one aspect of this and is not an adequate description of what the surgeon intends to do. Finnis et al assert that a surgeon performing craniotomy "resisting the undue influence of physical and causal factors that would dominate

---

[121] *Veritatis Splendor,* n. 78.
[122] Finnis et al, op. cit., pp. 22-3.

the perception of observers, could rightly say "No way do I intend to kill the baby" and "It is no part of my purpose to kill the baby." They say that the killing in this case is not brought about as a chosen means and thus is not the immediate object in the sense defined in *Veritatis Splendor*.[123]

I cannot see that there can be a separation between the moral description of the act and the clear psychological intent, which is to dismember the head in a way that is death dealing in itself not as a side effect. There is a false distinction being made between moral and psychological intent. The major problem in the Finnis et al analysis is that they permit a moral narrative that is psychologically strained, so strained as to be totally implausible as a way in which anyone would actually reason. The acting person who reasoned like that could only be self-deceiving.

The morally relevant description of the act is narrowing the head of the child by dismembering it. That may save the life of the mother, but the direct object is the dismembering, and that is synonymous with the death of the child.

There is a difference between this case and the types of cases for which double-effect reasoning ordinarily applies, where the death is clearly a side effect, such as bombing a military installation and killing citizens who happen to be in the vicinity, or removing a gravid cancerous uterus resulting in the loss of life of the child. In the case of dismembering a child to save the life of the mother, the death is integral to what is chosen rather than beside it. The death is synonymous with the act that is necessary to achieve the end of saving life. Someone who dismembers a child but describes their act according to the preferred consequence of saving life and not as a killing is deceiving themselves as to the nature of the act. A morally relevant feature is that the desired consequence is only part of the reality of what is deliberately chosen. Nevertheless, to say that in dismembering the child, which is clearly the immediate object, I did not intend the death is just plainly untrue. This case, it seems to me, is quite unlike removing the gravid but cancerous

---

[123] Ibid., p. 23.

uterus. In the latter case the act results in death but the act is clearly separable from the death in that the latter is a side effect and therefore beside the intention. Death is not a side effect of dismembering a baby, it is the main event.

There is a difference between attempting to remove the child by forceps delivery and causing the child's death in the process, on the one hand, and, on the other hand, deliberately dismembering the child, as Grisez has described it, in order to achieve removal. The difference is between what is the immediate object and what is truly a side effect. Thus I can accept dismembering the head of the child (and death) if it happens as a side effect of attempts to remove, but not where the procedure in the first instance involves dismembering the head as a step on the way to removal.

I disagree with Finnis et al when, in response to Kevin Flannery, they say that the relevant description of the act of dismembering the head would not involve killing the baby. Psychologically killing the baby would stand foremost as what the surgeon is doing in dismembering the head. On the other hand, if the surgeon attempted a forceps delivery in these circumstances and that resulted, or was likely or even certain to result, in dismemberment while trying to remove the child, that would be different from going in with a procedure to dismember the head of the child. The surgeon could consider the dismemberment to be a side effect of forceps delivery but not if the dismemberment was the immediate goal of the procedure, presumably with instruments designed to dismember rather than forceps.

Finnis et al analyse a case that would seem to bear upon this problem. In their case E, they refer to a farmer who castrates male calves in order to effect hormonal changes that will make them fatter and calmer. The authors say sterilizing is not a means or an end and hence is not part of the proposal to fatten the claves. The case, they argue, makes it clear that, depending on what one proposes to do and what one only accepts as a side effect, one can be doing either of two acts different in kind even though everything about one's behaviour and the observable context is the same. The point seems to turn on their claim that sterilization is not essential to the goal of fattening the calves but is a side effect.

The removing of the testes, which is what the sterilization procedure involves, results in the loss of a source of hormones and that loss causes fattening and calmness. The loss of fertility is also an effect of the loss of the testes as they produce sperm. Finnis et al would claim that the loss of capacity to produce sperm (sterilization) is a side effect because it is not part of the proposal but foreseen or permitted. I struggle with this. I am unable to separate conceptually removing testes and removing the capacity to produce sperm. Generating sperm is what testes do. Psychologically it would seem to me that the procedure is to sterilize, because sterilizing causes fattening and calming. Unmanageable stallions are gelded for similar reasons. But the gelding could not be considered a side effect. Gelding is the event that usually produces the manageability and anyone who told a farmer that gelding was not sterilization would risk being laughed at or pitied.

Finnis et al argue that their account differs from previous accounts that have led the Magisterium to find teaching that supports craniotomy to be unsafe. The difference lies in their rejection of the position that they attribute to Henry Davis SJ and which appears in most accounts of double-effect reasoning:[124] that the good effect must follow at least as immediately and directly as the evil effect. It seems that this principle is an attempt to capture, in part, how it is that the evil in the act is indirect. It is a notion that extends beyond direct lines of causality; that is, the Davis principle does not claim that the impermissible evil is a means to the good, but rather that it precedes or is more immediate than the good.

This is, of course, the case with craniotomy. The dismembering and thus the death precede and are more immediate than the removal of the child that results in the saving of life. The latter is secondary to the procedure to dismember. Finnis et al argue that the traditional principle (the Davis principle) is a mistake, referring to the soldier who throws himself on a grenade to save others. We applaud his heroism,

---

[124] Ibid., pp. 19-20.

but his body being destroyed is more immediate than the grenade not doing injury or as much injury to his fellows.

There is, however, a substantial difference between the soldier's heroism and my actions were I to have thrown the soldier on top of the grenade to save others. I am not sure that our acceptance of the heroism has anything to do with claiming that his act is indirect killing. As a psychological narrative, would it be indirect killing in the case of my throwing him on to the grenade? I think not.

As examples of this reasoning, Finnis et al then cite the mention in *Evangelium Vitae* of double-effect reasoning in relation to pain relief and refusal of burdensome life support where death is a side effect. *EV* says that in those cases the death is not willed or sought. But both of those cases are quite different from Finnis et al's account in which the evil is more immediate than the good. In the *EV* instances, the pain relief and the lessening of the burden of treatment are more immediate than the death. If in fact the death was expected to precede lessening of the burden or the relief of pain, then death would appear psychologically to be the immediate object (rather than the lessening of the burden). Rather than demonstrating their narrative of the moral act the *EV* text would seem to indicate difference from it.

There is something of a connection between the Finnis et al account and proportionalism in that both seem to override the significance of direct killing. In Finnis et al, the moral narrative overrides the psychological narrative of direct killing. In the case of McCormick, the evil of direct killing is overridden by a commensurate reason. It seems to me that Finnis et al's account strengthens McCormick's position by substituting a moral narrative in place of the psychological narrative. In both narratives, what is psychologically direct killing is not considered to be morally relevant.

The issue of proportionalism is addressed in the encyclical *Veritatis Splendor*. The precise goal or purpose of *Veritatis Splendor* is to recall "certain fundamental truths of Catholic doctrine which, in the present circumstances, risk being distorted or denied."[125]

---

[125] *Veritatis Splendor*, n. 4.

Pope John Paul II refers to "false solutions, linked in particular to an inadequate understanding of the object of moral action." He argues that such false solutions lead to a denial of the existence of "intrinsically evil acts." These last are particularly linked with certain "teleological ethical theories (proportionalism, consequentialism)."[126]

Pope John Paul II rejects as erroneous any theory *"which holds that it is impossible to qualify as morally evil according to its species – its 'object' – the deliberate choice of certain kinds of behaviour or specific acts, apart from a consideration of the intention for which the choice is made or the totality of the foreseeable consequences of that act for all persons concerned."*[127]

In my view this teaching not only excludes proportionalism, it also excludes Finnis et al's separation of a moral narrative from the psychological narrative and their rejection of the time-honoured claim that in double-effect reasoning the evil must not be more immediate than the good sought. The latter, it seems to me, reflects accurately the psychological reality and the moral narrative cannot rightly be separated from the psychological reality. If I deliberately dismember someone's head, I mean to kill them.

The Pope reaffirmed that there exists "moral commandments ... which prohibit always and without exception *intrinsically evil acts.*"[128] An up-to-date version of double-effect reasoning might therefore be expressed as:

1. The immediate object of the act must be capable of being directed towards God and must therefore not violate a divine commandment or otherwise destroy a basic human good.
2. The agent may not positively will the bad effect as a means to the good end but may permit it as a side effect of what is positively willed. If he or she could attain the good effect without the bad effect, he or she should do so.
3. The bad effect must not be directly willed but may be

---
[126] Ibid., n. 75.
[127] Ibid., n 79.
[128] Ibid., n. 115.

permitted as being indirectly voluntary. For the evil to be indirect and thus permissible, the good effect must flow from the action at least as immediately as the bad effect.

4. The bad effect must not be disproportionate to the good effect, nor unjust.

3.6 Fundamental Option

An attractive approach to Christian ethics was taken by Karl Rahner, who related moral theology to his accounts of prayer and grace. Rahner was a *peritus* at the Second Vatican Council and both prolific and enormously influential.

Rahner focused on our relationship to God and referred to what he calls the "fundamental option" in which a person is in friendship with God in his or her whole being, not just by a particular choice or act. Recognising the imperfect nature of our knowledge of our selves and of the nature of our relationships and our acts, adherents of the fundamental option conclude that no ordinary decision can be such as to reverse the basic direction of our friendship with God, as the individual's choosing ordinarily lacks the necessary understanding to choose to reject God at that deep level at which the friendship with God is formed.[129]

In a similar vein, Joseph Fuchs SJ, distinguishes between the ordinary level of freedom of moral acts and a deeper level about which he writes:

> Basic freedom, on the other hand, denotes a still more fundamental, deeper-rooted freedom, not immediately accessible to psychological investigation. This is the freedom that enables us not only to decide freely on particular acts and aims but also,

---

[129] Karl Rahner SJ, *Foundations of Christian Faith: An Introduction to the Idea of Christianity,* trans. William V. Dych, (New York: Seabury Press, 1978) pp. 93-106; Karl Rahner SJ, "Theology of Freedom," *Theological Investigations,* Vol 6, *Concerning Vatican Council II,* trans. Karl-H. and Boniface Kruger, (Baltimore: Helicon, 1969), pp. 190-93.

by means of these, to determine ourselves totally as persons and not merely in any particular area of behaviour. It is clear that man's freedom of choice and his basic freedom are not simply two different psychological freedoms. As a person, man is free. But this freedom can, of course, be considered under different aspects. A man can, in one and the same act, choose the object of his choice (freedom of choice) and by so doing determine himself as a person (basic freedom).

Rahner recognizes self-determination and moral responsibility in free choices and, seemingly accurately, represents the importance of free choice in the Christian tradition. However his theory of fundamental option is not so much about moral principles but theological anthropology; for him, fundamental freedom of the will corresponds to the preconceptual orientation of intellect to God.[130] He identifies freedom with the commandment to love, which may characterise the underlying orientation of the person in his or her friendship with God such that this love at that deep level may transcend the person's choices with respect to the other commandments.[131]

Germain Grisez summarises the attraction of fundamental option as appealing to:

- a rejection of legalism that requires correct performance with respect to individual acts, such as the Decalogue, with the focus instead on the person's general orientation of friendship with God;
- the Christian life considered as a unified and developing whole, rather than on particular choices considered in isolation;
- an explanation that people can act out of character at times without permanently changing their character and thus

---

[130] Karl Rahner SJ, "Theology of Freedom," *Theological Investigations*, Vol 6, *Concerning Vatican Council II*, trans. Karl-H. and Boniface Kruger, (Baltimore: Helicon, 1969), pp. 178-86.
[131] Karl Rahner SJ, *Theological Investigations, Vol 5, Later Writings*, trans. Karl-H. Kruger, (Baltimore: Helicon 1966) pp. 445-51.

their basic orientation towards God.¹³²

Fundamental Option may thus be adopted as a very comforting theory that allows us to attach less importance to individual acts because the focus is on the deeper, underlying relationship.

Pope John Paul II addressed this matter in the encyclical *Veritatis Splendor* (nos. 66-70), in which he explained that the theory is contrary to the teaching of Scripture itself, which sees the fundamental option as a genuine choice of freedom and links that choice profoundly to particular acts. This is the meaning of the divine law and evident in the Decalogue. The commandments so express God's love for us and teach us how to love that violating a commandment is an act against love of God or neighbour.

It is true that we can make a fundamental choice that gives purpose and direction to our lives and through that choice, with the help of God's grace, we can follow God's call. However, following that call is actually exercised in the particular choices of specific actions through which we conform ourselves to God's Word. The Pope states:

> ...the so-called fundamental option, to the extent that it is distinct from a generic intention and hence one not yet determined in such a way that freedom is obligated, is always brought into play through conscious and free decisions. Precisely for this reason, it is revoked when man engages his freedom in conscious decisions to the contrary, with regard to morally grave matter.¹³³

---

[132] Germain Grisez, "The Distinction Between Grave and Light Matter", in his *The Way of the Lord Jesus, Volume 2, Christian Moral Principles*, (Chicago: Franciscan Herald Press, 1983).
[133] *Veritatis Splendor*, n. 67.

3.7 A Natural Law Ethic

3.7.1 Introduction

St Paul claims that even pagans know God's law because it is written in their hearts. This is generally referred to as "natural law". We can thus appeal to natural law rather than to revealed religion on matters of public policy. There are however tensions about what natural law is, its sources, and its teleology. One such tension is over a distinction between *synderesis* and *anamnesis,* which may be characterised in terms of a distinction between nature and grace and a distinction between *a priori* or *a posteriori* moral knowledge. A second significant tension is over teleology and the difference on that issue separates those who treat natural law anthropocentrically from those who treat it theocentrically. That distinction affects the characterisation of the basic human goods. This section examines the effects those differences have on natural law approaches to evangelization in the public forum of our secular societies, focussing particularly on the challenge of defending the Pauline Principle which is fundamental to a natural law approach but not well understood or accepted in secular discussion. Finally the section draws some conclusions, from that discussion of the sources of natural law and defending the Pauline Principle, about the nature of the task of moral evangelisation in the public forum of western secularism.

3.7.2 Synderesis and Anamnesis

In his encyclical *Evangelium Vitae*, Pope John Paul II affirmed the right to life in terms of a natural law that results both from reason and from grace:

> Even in the midst of difficulties and uncertainties, every person sincerely open to truth and goodness can, by the light of reason and the hidden action of grace, come to recognise in the natural law written in the heart (cf Rom 2:14-15) the sacred value of human life from its very beginning until its end, and can affirm

the right of every human being to have this primary good respected...[134]

The contribution of divine grace and reason to our natural law is something of a tension in our tradition.

Natural law approaches to morality have in common the claim that there are objective moral grounds for knowing what is morally good and bad. One of the tensions over this knowledge is whether it is a *priori* or *a posteriori*. Those who follow Augustine may claim that it is *a priori* because placed directly by God from the outset, and in that sense "written in their hearts". Others may follow St. Thomas Aquinas in holding that it is *a posteriori* knowledge, believing that God gave us the capacity to reason and that we can gain knowledge of right and wrong by applying reason to our experiences of our human nature.

Two crucial concepts about which there are differences of opinion are "synderesis" and 'anamnesis". Synderesis is the natural or innate ability of the mind to know the first principles of ethics and moral reasoning. The concept is both intellectual and volitional and it fits those versions of natural law that argue for the self evidence of the basic human goods in our experience of our human reality and our relationships and thus as the basis for forming conscience as a reasoning process guided by that experience of the basic human goods. In other words, synderesis is *a posteriori* and reflects a confidence in human reasoning which may be based on us being made in the image and likeness of God and thus possessing the capacity to the intellectual and volitional capacity to reason in this way and to recognise goodness and to choose it.

However the present Pope, then as Cardinal Ratzinger criticised the notion of synderesis insisting that the concept of anamnesis better reflects what is meant by the Pauline passage and the law written in our hearts. Cardinal Ratzinger writes:

> The love of God is not founded on a discipline imposed on us from outside, but is constitutively established in us as the

---

[134] *Evangelium Vitae*, n. 2.

capacity and necessity of our rational nature." Basil speaks in terms of "the spark of divine love which has been hidden in us," an expression which was to become important in medieval mysticism. In the spirit of Johannine theology, Basil knows that love consists in keeping the commandments. For this reason, the spark of love which has been put into us by the Creator, means this: "We have received interiorly beforehand the capacity and disposition for observing all divine commandments ... These are not something imposed from without." Referring everything back to its simple core, Augustine adds: "We could never judge that one thing is better than another if a basic understanding of the good had not already been instilled in us."[135]

Cardinal Ratzinger claims that conscience consists in the fact that something like an original memory of the good and true has been implanted in us, that there is an inner ontological tendency within man, who is created in the likeness of God, toward the divine. From its origin, man's being resonates with some things and clashes with others. He writes:

> This anamnesis of the origin, which results from the godlike constitution of our being is not a conceptually articulated knowing, a store of retrievable contents. It is so to speak an inner sense, a capacity to recall, so that the one whom it addresses, if he is not turned in on himself, hears its echo from within. He sees: "That's it! That is what my nature points to and seeks.[136]

This difference between synderesis and anamnesis has serious implications for evangelization in Bioethics and in all areas of public policy. If we take the view that there is an innate moral sense, then our task of moral evangelization is to so present the truth that our audience recalls that innate knowledge, despite the ravages of sin having so dimmed that moral sense. If we take the view that moral knowledge

---

[135] Joseph Cardinal Ratzinger, "Conscience and Truth", presented at the 10th Workshop for Bishops February, 1991, Dallas, Texas, http://www.ewtn.com/library/curia/ratzcons.htm (accessed August 6, 2010).
[136] Ibid., Section 3.

is attained through applying our inherited capacity to reason to our experience, then our task of evangelization is to seek to convince by building an argument for our principles through pure reason.

3.7.3 Teleology

The distinction between synderesis and anamnesis may also impact the way in which natural law reasoning is undertaken particularly in relation to teleology because anamnesis is obviously theocentric rather than anthropocentric. Nevertheless, St Thomas outlines an approach based on synderesis that is still theocentric. For St Thomas the true ultimate end of all human beings is God alone, attained by the beatific vision.[137] St Thomas had not moved far from St Augustine, who favoured anamnesis over synderesis. For St Thomas, God remained central to his approach to understanding human nature and the natural law. However some contemporary natural law theorists have adopted an anthropocentric teleology.

Natural law in Catholic thinking is usually sourced to St Thomas. In recent times it has had its defenders in what has come to be called "New Natural Law" which was initiated by Germain Grisez in the 1960s and his collaborators include Joseph Boyle, John Finnis, and Olaf Tollfeson. Others who have joined the ranks more recently include Robert P George, Patrick Lee, Fr Peter Ryan SJ, Gerald Bradley, William May, Christian Brugger and Christopher Tollefson.

Contemporary new natural law theorists (NNLT), such as Germain Grisez, argue that our ultimate end is not the beatific vision but a state of affairs that includes all persons with whom or for whose sake we can act, including God, with whose creative activity we cooperate in pursuing basic goods. We thus seek integral communal fulfilment by pursuing the basic goods and avoiding evil.[138] Thus synderesis for new natural law is even more distant from anamnesis than it was for St Thomas for whom it retained its theocentrism.

---

[137] St Thomas Aquinas, *Summa Theologiae* 1–2, q. 1, aa. 1, 4, 6. and q. 2, a. 8, c.
[138] Germain Grisez, "The True and Ultimate End of Human Beings: The Kingdom, Not God Alone", *Theological Studies,* Vol 69, 2008, pp. 38-61.

The NNLT approach may be attractive because it better suits the challenge of secular discussion because it is anthropocentric and religion becomes just one of the basic human goods. The theocentrism of St Thomas leaves us with less to say to those who do not believe.

For a Christian philosopher to ignore what has been revealed to us in the Scriptures and what has developed in our tradition would be foolish. However we may be inclined to do so when engaged in secular debate in which others do not share our beliefs and culture. That is to say in public discussion we may be more inclined to offer a justification for what we believe in a way that may persuade others rather than to appeal to the "spark of the divine" within them that has us recall knowledge of good and evil. A politician wishing to explain why he wishes to vote to protect human life, is unlikely to do the latter.

Alasdair MacIntyre is a contemporary defender of new natural law approaches. MacIntyre makes a distinction between moral truth and moral justification in response to relativism. He argues that moral truth exists independently of a justification offered from any particular standpoint or view. However to give an account of moral truth we need to give an account of the existence of pluralism despite moral truth. Thus in considering all the rival justifications that are offered, he suggests that which has the greatest claim to truth is that which has moved furthest from initial local, partial and one-sided points of view towards a type of understanding – and in the case of the moral life a type of practice – freed in some significant way from the limitations of such partiality and one-sidedness and possessed of the resources which would enable it to explain, in the light of the comprehension thus achieved, just why it is that they appear otherwise from the limited perspectives of those local, partial, and one-sided standpoints which limitations have now been transcended.[139]

MacIntyre argues that the natural law tradition has attained that goal. In general, theories of natural law are teleological. That is to say

---

[139] Alasdair MacIntyre, "Moral Relativism, Truth and Justification" in his *The Task of Philosophy, Vol 1* (New York: Cambridge University Press, 2006) pp. 52-73.

they propose a goal or goal for human beings and then discuss how that goal may be attained. Natural law has a positive, even optimistic, understanding of human nature and the power of reason.[140]

I offer a summary of Grisez's account on natural law here as a possible approach to justification of a moral view which may still be standing in comparison to other views subjected to the approach that Macintyre proposes of excluding local, partial, and one-sided standpoints and able to explain the mistakes that other views may make in the latter respects.

Grisez follows St Thomas in saying that according to St. Thomas, the very first principle of practical reasoning in general is: *The good is to be done and pursued; the bad is to be avoided.*[141] By this is not meant explicitly moral good and evil. Rather "good" in this context simply means that which is intelligibly worthwhile. Applying Macintyre's notion of justification devoid of any particular standpoint, this principle seems self evident, it reflects what the words "good" and "evil" mean, and they do not at this point contain a particular notion of the good that might be derived from an individual standpoint. To say the opposite, "evil is to be done and good avoided" would seem to be contradictory. As Grisez expresses it, the first principle of practical reasoning articulates the intrinsic, necessary relationship between human goods and appropriate actions bearing upon them.[142]

> "As it comes from the hand of God, all creation is good. "God saw everything that he had made, and behold, it was very good" (Gn 1.31). Even things touched by sin can be redeemed, for their original goodness is not wholly corrupted. "For everything created by God is good, and nothing is to be rejected if it is received with thanksgiving; for then it is consecrated by the word of God and prayer" (1 Tm 4.4–5). Made in God's image, human persons as created, fleshly beings are completely good."[143]

---

[140] Ray Campbell in lectures to graduate students at the John Paul II Institute January 2006.
[141] St Thomas Aquinas *Summa Theologica* 1–2, q. 94, a. 2.
[142] Germain Grisez, *The Way of the Lord Jesus, Vol 1, Christian Moral Principles,* "Natural Law" and the Chapter 7 "Fundamental Principles of Morality", 7 F n. 6.
[143] Ibid., 5 A 1.

This assumption that all creation, and specifically all human beings, are good may be challenged, firstly by those who do not believe in a Creator. Some such as Ronald Dworkin, accept it, but only as a religious belief and hence in his view not properly the subject of law and public policy. The assumption that human beings are good may be defended on other grounds. A moral theory that did not accept the worthwhileness of human beings would be possible, but would seem to be somehow self defeating.

Grisez defines "bad" in terms of the negative of good: "The bad is present in what is distorted, damaged, and corrupted in creatures. The badness of what is bad is precisely the distorting, damaging, or corrupting factor. This factor is a privation, a real lack of something which should be present and perfect."[144]

From his notion of the good we can derive the assumption that a goal of practical reason is the well-being of happiness or well-being of people. On that basis Grisez invokes the notion of "fullness of being" to explain what the basic human goods are. These are not instrumental to human well-being, such as food or property, but those goods that are actually constitutive of human fullness of being. Because the goods are constitutive of fullness of being human, for us a basic human good provides a reason for choosing and acting that requires no further justification. Basic human goods perfect human beings and contribute to their communities.[145]

Grisez distinguishes between reflexive or substantive good. Reflexive goods are both reasons for choosing and are in part defined in terms of choosing and they include:
 (1) self-integration, which is harmony among all the parts of a person which can be engaged in freely chosen action;
 (2) practical reasonableness or authenticity, which is harmony among moral reflection, free choices, and their execution;
 (3) justice and friendship, which are aspects of the interpersonal communion of good persons freely choosing to act in

---
[144] Ibid.
[145] Ibid., 5 D n. 11.

harmony with one another; and

(4) religion or holiness, which is harmony with God, found in the agreement of human individual and communal free choices with God's will.[146]

The reflexive goods also can be called "existential" or "moral," since they fulfill human subjects and interpersonal groups in the existential dimension of their being.[147]

The other three categories of basic human goods fulfill persons in the other three dimensions of their being. These goods can be called "nonreflexive" or "substantive," since they are not defined in terms of choosing, and they provide reasons for choosing which can stand by themselves. These are:

(1) life itself, including health, physical integrity, safety, and the handing on of life to new persons;
(2) knowledge of various forms of truth and appreciation of various forms of beauty or excellence; and
(3) activities of skillful work and of play, which in their very performance enrich those who do them.[148]

Not everyone agrees with this analysis of the basic human goods. Some are troubled by Grisez's teleology which makes the good of religion just one of the basic human goods in pursuit of integral human fulfilment, rather than the pursuit of communion with God. But more of this later.

In his encyclical *Veritatis Splendor*, Pope John Paul II asserts that it is in the light of the dignity of the human person – a dignity which must be affirmed for its own sake – that reason grasps the specific moral value of certain goods towards which the person is naturally inclined. And since the human person cannot be reduced to a freedom which is self-designing, but entails a particular spiritual and bodily structure, the primordial moral requirement of loving and respecting the person as an end, and never as a mere means, also implies, by its

---
[146] Ibid.
[147] Ibid.
[148] Ibid.

very nature, respect for certain fundamental goods, without which one would fall into relativism and arbitrariness.[149]

There is a congruence between Grisez's practicable reasonableness or natural law and Scripture. Jesus taught that we should love God and love our neighbour and keep the ten commandments.[150] Pope John Paul II writes that the different commandments of the Decalogue are really only so many reflections of the one commandment about the good of the person, at the level of the many different goods which characterize his identity as a spiritual and bodily being in relationship with God, with his neighbour and with the material world.[151]

The *Catechism of the Catholic Church* teaches that the Ten Commandments are part of God's Revelation. At the same time, they teach us man's true humanity. They shed light on the essential duties, and so indirectly on the fundamental rights, inherent in the nature of the human person.[152]

According to Pope John Paul II, the commandments are meant to safeguard *the good* of the person, the image of God, by protecting the *goods* that are constitutive of the fullness of being of a human person. "You shall not murder; You shall not commit adultery; You shall not steal; You shall not bear false witness" are moral rules formulated in terms of prohibitions. These negative precepts express with particular force the ever urgent need to protect human life, the communion of persons in marriage, private property, truthfulness and people's good name. The commandments thus represent the basic condition for love of neighbour.[153]

He writes:

> Judgments about morality cannot be made without taking into consideration whether or not the deliberate choice of a specific kind of behaviour is in conformity with the dignity and integral

---

[149] *Veritatis Splendor*, n. 48.
[150] Matthew 5-7.
[151] *Veritatis Splendor*, n.13.
[152] *Catechism of the Catholic Church*, No. 2070.
[153] *Veritatis Splendor*, n.13.

vocation of the human person. Every choice always implies a reference by the deliberate will to the goods and evils indicated by the natural law as goods to be pursued and evils to be avoided. In the case of the positive moral precepts, prudence always has the task of verifying that they apply in a specific situation, for example, in view of other duties which may be more important or urgent. But the negative moral precepts, those prohibiting certain concrete actions or kinds of behaviour as intrinsically evil, do not allow for any legitimate exception. They do not leave room, in any morally acceptable way, for the "creativity" of any contrary determination whatsoever. Once the moral species of an action prohibited by a universal rule is concretely recognized, the only morally good act is that of obeying the moral law and of refraining from the action which it forbids.[154]

Thus the structure of natural law in the way in which it has been explained by Grisez and others in the tradition of St Thomas Aquinas begins with the logical principle that *the good is to be done and pursued; the bad is to be avoided.* Bad is understood as the negative of good.

The assumption is made that human beings are good, which for believers is understood in terms of our being made in the image and likeness of God, but it is an assumption that has broad acceptance in that for us to believe otherwise would be self defeating.

That goodness is then understood in terms of the fullness of our being as human beings and the goods that are constitutive of the fullness of being. It thus follows that we should pursue those basic human goods and avoid acting against them.

We can readily understand this notion of natural law as the "law written in our hearts" of which St Paul wrote because it is based on the *imago dei* and thus fits within what Cardinal Ratzinger referred to as "anamnesis', our recall of our essential goodness in being made in God's image and likeness, the "spark of divine love" within us by which we have been given the capacity to recognise the goods and the

---

[154] *Veritatis Splendor*, n. 67.

disposition for observing all divine commandments.[155]

An important aspect of natural law morality therefore is that it explains that the divine law is not arbitrary. The Decalogue protects the fullness of human being and thus gives meaning to the commandment to love God and love one another:

Jesus was asked by the rich young man, "Which is the greatest commandment in the law?" And Jesus said to him, 'You shall love the Lord your God with all your heart, and with all your soul, and with all your mind. This is the great and first commandment. And a second is like it, You shall love your neighbour as yourself. On these two commandments depend all the law and the prophets."[156]

This is consistent with the Old Testament attitude to the Law: "observe all these laws ... so as to be happy..."[157]

The natural law tradition goes back at least as far as Aristotle and the Stoics and the Old Testament, and is consistent with the fulfillment of the law in Christ. The aim is to respect goodness in order to participate in the fullness of life. We choose the good and avoid evil not as the price for getting into heaven, but because it is essentially what is good for us. God as unqualified goodness can be seen as the source of the goodness of all the basic goods. Fulfilment through instantiations of human goods can be seen as participation in divine goodness – in that sense, God can be seen as ultimate end.[158]

The first principle that we choose good and avoid evil and the explanation of what is good and what is evil gives us a basic structure for morality that does not require single standpoint assumptions. It is on those grounds that Macintyre can claim that natural law is a candidate for being the most justifiable of alternative moral theories.

In Grisez's account he also includes what he calls "modes of responsibility". He writes that the modes of responsibility specify – "pin down" – the primary moral principle (choose good and avoid evil) by excluding as immoral those actions which involve willing in

---
[155] Joseph Cardinal Ratzinger, "Conscience and Truth", op. cit.
[156] Matthew 22:36.
[157] Deuteronomy 6:24.
[158] *Veritatis Splendor*, n. 13.

certain specific ways inconsistent with a will toward integral human fulfillment.[159]

Grisez's eight modes of responsibility[160] are:

1. One should not be deterred by felt inertia from acting for intelligible goods.
2. One should not be pressed by enthusiasm or impatience to act individualistically for intelligible goods.
3. One should not choose to satisfy an emotional desire except as part of one's pursuit and/or attainment of an intelligible good other than the satisfaction of the desire itself.
4. One should not choose to act out of an emotional aversion except as part of one's avoidance of some intelligible evil other than the inner tension experienced in enduring that aversion.
5. One should not, in response to different feelings toward different persons, willingly proceed with a preference for anyone unless the preference is required by intelligible goods themselves.
6. One should not choose on the basis of emotions which bear upon empirical aspects of intelligible goods (or bads) in a way which interferes with a more perfect sharing in the good or avoidance of the bad.
7. One should not be moved by hostility to freely accept or choose the destruction, damaging, or impeding of any intelligible human good.
8. One should not be moved by a stronger desire for one instance of an intelligible good to act for it by choosing to destroy, damage, or impede some other instance of an intelligible good.[161]

I do not want to explore the individual modes of responsibility here,

---

[159] Grisez, op. cit., 7 G n.2.
[160] Grisez's three volumes of *The Way of the Lord Jesus* and the modes of responsibility are explained at: http://www.twotlj.org/G-1-8-S.html (accessed August 6, 2010).
[161] Grisez, op. cit. Vol 1, Chapter 8 G.

except that I think that they have a bearing on the notion of virtue.

The virtues are dispositions to goodness and the vices are dispositions to badness. A good moral character or personality is shaped by our moral education and experiences by which we learn to recognise and to choose good and avoid evil. Virtue thus has an existential meaning in that we form it and reinforce it by our decisions.

As Grisez explains the relationship, like the modes of responsibility, virtues are not concerned with specific kinds of acts. Virtues are aspects of personality as a whole when all the other dimensions of the self are integrated with morally good commitments.

> Commitments establish one's existential identity; a whole personality integrated with a morally good self is virtuous. Since such a personality is formed by choices which are in accord with the first principle of morality and the modes of responsibility, the virtues embody the modes. In other words, the modes of responsibility shape the existential self of a good person, this self shapes the whole personality, and so good character embodies and expresses the modes.[162]

Thus the natural law in Church teaching reflects an openness to all the basic human goods constitutive of human flourishing and the pursuit of a coherent set of goods in a reasonable way. We may choose to do this in different ways depending on our aptitudes, opportunities and life circumstances. There is no one prescribed way of being a good person.

Pope John Paul teaches that

> Acting is morally good when the choices of freedom are in conformity with man's true good and thus express the voluntary ordering of the person towards his ultimate end...[163]

Our capacity for goodness is grasped by reason in the very being of a human being, as a matter of the integral truth about human nature, including our natural inclinations, motivations and purpose for existing.

---
[162] Grisez, op. cit., Chpt 7, H, 3.
[163] *Veritatis Splendor,* n. 72.

The Pope goes on to say it is precisely these which are the contents of the natural law. The ordered complex of 'personal goods' which serve the 'good of the person' are the good of the person tending toward perfection. These are the goods safeguarded by the commandments which, according to St Thomas, contain the whole natural law.[164]

A criticism of new natural law is that the end is not the beatific vision but a state of affairs that includes all persons with whom or for whose sake we can act, including God, with whose creative activity we cooperate in pursuing basic goods. In thus seeking integral communal fulfilment by pursuing the basic goods and avoiding evil,[165] the place of God in our lives appears to be just another good rather than the primary goal. As noted earlier this is a difference between Grisez and Aquinas.

Relegating God to an also ran status in our purposes does seem a little odd. However in practice the difference between, on the one hand, seeking fulfilment in communion with God and therefore also seeking communion with human beings made in God's image and likeness and loved by God, and, on the other, seeking fulfilment in communion with all persons including God, may not amount to much. We end up basically doing and pursuing the same range of goods and avoiding the same evils.

I guess one of the advantages of Grisez's schema is that, in placing human fulfilment through communion with other persons first, it is more open to those who do not believe but, like Aristotle and the Stoics, can accept the fundamental ideas of human beings as social beings and their fulfilment being in each other by the pursuit of human goodness, with religious belief being basically whatever is made of it by the individual including, perhaps non-belief for those who do not believe. Grisez's schema permits dialogue with believers and non-believers alike rather than being dependant on belief in God.

Certainly in the task of seeking a universal ethic to apply to medicine

---

[164] *Veritatis Splendor*, n. 79.
[165] Germain Grisez "The True and Ultimate End of Human Beings: The Kingdom, Not God Alone", *Theological Studies*, Vol 69, 2008: pp. 38-61.

and public policy, Grisez's approach may be more flexible. On the other hand it is open to the criticisms above that Cardinal Ratzinger made of philosophical approaches that added Jesus as a kind of "crowning". It also leaves the theological virtues in some kind of limbo.

However, the difference between Grisez and Aquinas on the matter of our teleology, may not be without consequence for our assessments of the nature of a moral act.

3.8 Virtue Ethics

There are different concepts of virtue. Some have a strong moral content and are considered to be thick notions of virtue such as those espoused by Plato and Aristotle.

For Platonist moral theorists, their concept of the virtuous citizen is linked to a political ideal of citizenship enjoined by reason – the set of virtues is internally compatible and causally related to citizenship. The virtues are those aspects of character that are needed for someone to be a good citizen. By acting virtuously I act in ways that tend toward the good of my community. So someone who recognises the needs of others and aims to fulfil their needs practises the virtue of justice, which is an important element of relationship in a just society. Someone who is courageous in seeking to pursue the goods necessary for a community exhibits a character trait that is important for the society. Someone who is able to manage or moderate his or her sexual or other inclinations for the purpose of achieving good relationships displays the virtue of temperance which is also important for the members of a community to have.

For Aristotelians the virtue of a thing is determined by its overall nature and purpose for existence. A virtue is that state of a thing that constitutes its peculiar essence and enables it to perform its function well – in humans, the activity of reason and of rationally ordered habits. Thus virtue may be recognised not just as a disposition necessary for being a citizen in a community, as the Platonists would have it, but may also be a disposition that tends to make our life go well. In other words, it is about our individual fulfilment. It is thus a causal notion in which we are disposed to recognise and choose the goods that are constitute of human fulfilment, and to avoid evil. The virtue of truth-telling protects the pursuit and sharing of knowledge, and is thus related to the good of knowledge. The virtues of chastity, temperance and fidelity involve the integration of sexuality into the fullness of the human person and tend to protect parenthood and nurturing of children and the loving relationships between persons, but more than that, it may be argued that, in possessing those virtues, we may in fact be happy in ourselves because those virtues tend towards the fullness of our own being and not just our community.

Post-modernism tends to treat the notion of virtue as a thin concept, merely as desirable characteristics. That is, a virtue is a characteristic that is met with approval by many or most people in our community. In that case, it is not a rational notion in the sense of being causally related to a theory about what is good and evil, and it is subject to differing views of the person and what is to be approved or disapproved.

Virtue is therefore a concept that may be affected by the moral views of a community and the circumstances of that community. For the ancient Greek writer Homer, virtue meant excellence in the standards of the time. For a man, that meant having the attributes of an heroic warrior king: fleet of foot, strong of arm, clear-sighted and capable in leadership and military tactics.

For the philosopher Immanuel Kant, virtue is the strength of one's will to fulfil one's duties in the face of obstacles. Thus one is virtuous when one's will predominates over one's natural inclinations. This differs from an Aristotelian view. For an Aristotelian, to act virtuously is not to act against inclination (as Kant would have it) but to act from inclination formed by the cultivation of the virtues on rational grounds. For the contemporary or neo-Aristotelians, virtues are the attitudes, habits, dispositions, willingness that can be justified as reasonable modes of response to the opportunities which intelligence makes evident to us.[166]

---

[166] JN Finnis, *Fundamentals of Ethics* (Oxford, Oxford University Press, 1983), p. 56

Because of the causal relationship between virtue and the goods that constitute the fullness of human being, Aristotelian virtue is not rule-based, rather virtues relate to reason, to *eudaimonia* or having an objectively desirable life. Aristotle recognized the social nature of humanity – hence *eudaimonia* is to some extent dependant on good citizenship and what is necessary to be a good citizen (which might be relative to the existing social order or to a reasonable ideal of social order).

Aristotelian virtue includes the notion that moral virtues make possible ease, self-mastery, and joy in leading a morally good life. The virtuous person freely practices the good unimpeded by vice (dispositions toward evil). At the same time, the moral virtues are acquired by human effort and are the result and the source of morally good acts.

Once when travelling with one of my daughters and a friend in the car their conversation focused on one of their classmates whose character they attacked with adolescent stridency. I attempted to explore their attitude towards her, suggesting that in fact their attitude was one of envy rather than any great character deficit of their peer. Conversations of that nature seldom quite go as one might hope. But the thrust of what I wanted to say was that the emotion that they experienced would be better directed toward exploring why they felt inferior and what they might do to improve in areas in which they felt that way.

That response was in essence Aristotelian. The virtuous person is a happy person precisely because they shape their desires and their acts towards the pursuit of the good. In that sense they achieve self mastery and can be at ease with themselves and their circumstances.

The causal relationship between the goods of human fullness of being and what are often called the "Cardinal Virtues" are easily identified. They include:

- Wisdom (Prudence) – which disposes practical reason to discern good and to choose the rights means to achieve it;
- Justice – uprightness of conduct towards one's neighbour;

- Courage – firmness in difficulties in the pursuit of good;
- Temperance – which ensures the mastery of the will over instincts.

The Cardinal Virtues are upheld by most if not all societies, because if one lacked any one of them, one would find it very difficult to live in a community and one would in all probability be very miserable, and perhaps even mentally ill. One can appreciate the importance of the Cardinal Virtues by reflecting, for a moment, on what it would be like to not be able to recognise goodness, not be able to recognise the needs of others and to respond to them, to lack the courage to go out and face the community or the tasks that are necessary just to survive, or to lack control of one's base desires and instincts.

The fundamental question that underlies what virtues are is: What kind of person ought I to be? Logically it is prior to the question: What ought I to do? On the other hand, however, what I do determines the kind of person that I am.

In his book *The Ethics of Authenticity* the philosopher Charles Taylor argues that reasoning in morality is reasoning with someone else; it is a dialogue, and not a solitary activity. On that basis he argues that morality is essentially communitarian rather then individualist, and that individual choice needs "horizons of significance." A causal concept of virtue provides horizons of significance that relate to the fullness of being human through pursuing good and avoiding evil.

A thin concept of the human person and human community tends toward individualism and upholding autonomy as the highest value, and avoiding heteronomy (where we accept the rules of others). It sees us basically as survivors in the necessary evil of community.

A thick or rich notion of the human person and community is likely to focus on relationships and co-operation as being constitutive of who we are, and to embrace pursuing goods in common and having life plans influenced by the needs of others and a common humanitarian duty of care.

Some virtues that are a result of such a thick notion may include:

- respectfulness and fellow-feeling;
- prudence;
- courage and patience;
- temperance;
- justice, fairness and solidarity;
- liberality, mercy or rescue;
- fidelity;
- respect and gratitude;
- truthfulness;
- efficiency.

A thick notion would avoid vices such as:

- maleficience;
- infidelity;
- impiety;
- meanness;
- prodigality or inefficiency;
- cowardice;
- intemperateness;
- partiality or bigotry.

One of the puzzles for moral philosophy is the significance and derivation of what are called the "Theological Virtues" – faith, hope and love. It is often argued that these are not derivable from pure reason and that they are either recalled by us in faith through our origin in the image and likeness of Christ or learned through revelation in Holy Scripture.

For a Christian, faith is belief in God and in all that he has said and revealed to us. For a Catholic, faith includes belief in what the Church proposes for our belief. We accept the authority of the Church as appointed by Christ. Faith is a commitment of self to God, trusting in his infinite goodness, because he is truth itself. For this reason the believer seeks to know and do God's will.

The Catechism teaches that faith is a gift and remains in anyone who has not sinned against it; and that when it is deprived of hope and love, faith does not fully unite the believer to Christ and does not make him or her a living member of Christ's Body.[167]

St Augustine teaches that hope has for its object only what is good, and only what is future, and only what affects the person who entertains the hope.[168] The virtue of hope is linked to happiness by inspiring us, preventing discouragement, sustaining us at times of loss, and laying open our expectation of eternal happiness with God.

The practice of all the virtues is affected by love, which "binds everything together in perfect harmony;" it is the form of the virtues; it articulates and orders them among themselves; it is the source and the goal of their Christian practice. Human love connects us to God who is love.

An area that is highly relevant to a book on bioethics is a account of virtues in relation to being a health professional.

Post modernism may see the set of virtues of health professionals as being determined by social approval. However, someone who sees virtue in the context of practical reason will instead see the virtues causally as those character traits that are necessary to be a good health professional and hence shaped by the purposes, ends or teleology of medicine.

The first step would be to list the aims or purposes of medicine, perhaps including:

1. curing ill-health and or disease;
2. maintaining health;
3. preventing or at least slowing down the progress of disease;
4. maintaining or improving function or at least slowing the progress of disability;
5. preventing the development of disease or illness;
6. helping a patient in a holistic way to understand ill-health or disease and its treatment;
7. relieving or controlling uncomfortable or distressing symptoms;

---
[167] *Catechism of the Catholic Church* n. 1815.
[168] St Augustine, *The Enchiridion*, Ch. 8. n.71.

8. helping a patient and family to accept a prognosis of illness, disease, disability and eventually death.

The question about the necessary virtues of the health professionals then is about what is required for those ends to be attainable. We can certainly see a place for the cardinal virtues:

1. *prudence or wisdom* in determining what is good for the patient, taking into account not just the physical nature of illness and disease, but also the holistic effects on the patient in all his or her circumstances;
2. *temperance* in managing one's own inclinations, especially in circumstances in which the patient is particularly vulnerable, or is difficult or irritating or downright hostile and angry.
3. *courage* in undertaking treatments, such as surgery, that require confidence in the health professional's great skill and ability, especially in the usual circumstances of relative factual uncertainty and therefore the possibility of doing harm, and courage to communicate a terminal diagnosis or prognosis;
4. *justice* in managing the efficient use of relatively scarce resources and in making bedside rationing decisions that take into account not just what is due to this patient but also the needs of others.

Many other virtues are needed to service the above goals, such as:

5. *knowledge and skills* to be able to diagnose and treat competently
6. *piety* – respect for the health and medical authorities including colleagues and their judgements, but also respect for the elderly and their place in the community;
7. *ability to communicate* complex information in a way that can be understood by a lay person;
8. *counselling skills* including the ability to listen to the patient and his or her values and perceptions, and to respond sensitively;

9. *truthfulness* in communicating information
10. *respect for the person* – his or her worth, autonomy and privacy so that the patient continues to trust the health professional;

Beyond those, however, are the virtues needed to deal with the inevitable nature of suffering and death. Patients die and not all suffering can be relieved. That calls on reserves in health professionals for them to accept suffering and death. This may require the theological virtues of *faith, hope and charity*. There is much to consider in determining what is needed for someone to be a good health professional, including matters related to religious belief.

On this account, virtue is therefore a causal notion that relies on the teleology or goals of the role or function.

4
Religion in a Secular Society

4.1 Introduction

The Australian Human Rights Commission recently proposed that there be a law to protect religious freedom. This occurred at a time when, in Australia, we have witnessed attempts, by those who express an aggressive form of secularism, to exclude religious commentary from public debate. Adherents of this view seem to hold that the doctrine of the separation of Church and state is not, as the constitution provides, the protection of the Church and people of religious beliefs from government interference with religious belief and practice, but rather justifies the exclusion of all but atheistic, or at least agnostic, views from involvement in public debate. Aggressive secularism would thus seem to have emerged as a form of anti-religious radicalism and intolerance.

This chapter focuses on issues around defining secularism and what kind of a secular society Australia is, and what role or place religions and religious beliefs have in a pluralist society. It explores the place of religious commentary in public debate in a pluralist society, and the emergence of the secularist view that public policy can be shaped by insisting on neutrality in relation to matters of private morality and religious belief, a neutrality that therefore excludes religious moral beliefs from the realm of public policy formation and law. I argue that rather than representing neutrality, this view of secularism would seem to have emerged as a belief system in itself and therefore a partisan basis for policy formation.

I argue instead for tolerance of the many different beliefs found within Australia as a pluralist society, and respect for the right, and the obligation, of all citizens to seek to participate in and contribute to the processes that lead to the formation of public policy. I suggest that as a tolerant society, we should welcome all to public debate so that public policy may be formed on the basis of listening to the arguments and evaluating proposals on their merits. In that way not only the outcomes, but also the processes by which we attain those outcomes, may give expression to equal respect for the worth and dignity of each member of the human family, within his or her cultural or community context and as we seek to attain our shared goal of serving the common good of humanity.

4.2. A Secular Society

The judgement that we live in a secular society may reflect an historical aberration, a modern phenomenon, and largely an exclusively Western phenomenon. Though there are other States, such as Turkey, that are constitutionally secular (notwithstanding the recent judicial difficulties of Turkey's ruling AK Party with its Moslem identity).

The philosopher Charles Taylor in his recent book *A Secular Age*[169] suggests that a secular society may be one in which one can engage fully in politics without ever encountering God. Apart from some vestigial prayers on such an occasion as the opening of Parliament, now to be preceded by a welcome from the original owners of our land (or an occasional speech from a member of minority religious party who became elected through the vagaries of the system for electing upper chambers and inter-party dealing on preferences), Australian politics are basically secular according to Taylor's characterisation.

In another sense though, Australia is even more secular than the USA. In 2005, only 40 per cent of Australian marriages took place in

---

[169] Charles Taylor, "A Secular Age", (Cambridge: Harvard University Press, 2007).

the presence of a Minister of religion,[170] whereas in the USA, 40 per cent took place without a Minister of religion.[171] The USA, despite a rigorous separation of Church and State, is the Western society with the highest statistics for religious belief and practice. Formal religious practice in Australia is in decline. In that sense, a secular society may mean a society in which people are predominantly not religious by belief or practice, especially where that is considered in terms of attendance at formal religious observances. By that measure, Turkey, though constitutionally secular, would not be described as secular, given that the vast majority of the population is Muslim, with 95 per cent declaring their belief in a God and adopting religious practices.[172]

Taylor however identifies a third sense of secularism, by which he means the rise of secularism as an alternative form of belief.

A society thus may be secular in three senses: first, religion not being a part of public life, the so-called separation of Church and State; second, declining religious belief and practice; or third, secularism as an alternative belief form.

In Australia, we are experiencing the third of these – secularism emerging as an alternative belief form, and it appears as a very aggressive, exclusionist form of secularism that views religious belief and practice with arrogant intolerance and dismissiveness. This kind of secularist belief is characterised by attempts to exclude contributions to public discussion on the basis of a kind of bigotry that classifies the contributions of persons who are religious in a nominalist way. The view is summed up in the title of a recent conference convened by the Fabian Society on the topic: "Separating Church & State: Keeping God Out of Government."

---

[170] Australian Bureau of Statistics, *Marriages Australia 2005* Document No. 3306.0.55.001, http://www.abs.gov.au/ausstats/abs@.nsf/mf/3306.0.55.001, (Accessed, April 1, 2008).
[171] http://atheism.about.com/b/2006/01/27/religious-marriage-vs-civil-marriage.htm
[172] European Commission, "Social values, Science and Technology" Eurobarometer 2005 http://ec.europa.eu/public_opinion/archives/ebs/ebs_225_report_en.pdf (Accessed April 1, 2008).

That secularism can be its own belief system can be seen in the words of Friedrich Nietzsche when he described the origin of positive atheism "to be found in a wholly deliberate act of choice, an inverted act of faith, a truly religious commitment in reverse."[173]

The problem is that ideological secularists seemed to have colonised the word "secular" to their own ends. In its origins, "secular" referred to the affairs of the world, that is, the governance of worldly affairs. Historically it had nothing to do with any idea of God being absent from the world, but was a recognition that the Church governs herself in the matters proper to herself and the State governs itself in the matters proper to itself without either institution as an institution usurping what is proper to each realm.[174]

It has, however, become no longer possible to use the term "secular" in its original meaning, as it has been taken over by those for whom it denotes a religious observance of an atheistic belief system or at the very least, an agnostic one, to the exclusion of any form of theism. In the age in which we live it might be better to use terms that are more properly descriptive of an inclusive multi-cultural, pluralist society in which everyone participates without discrimination as to race religion, class or cultural background. We ought perhaps to use the word "pluralism" to mean what was originally meant by "secularism." A pluralist society is one that is tolerant of a wide range of belief systems, inclusive of all persons whatever their beliefs or cultural background. In that way we would be taking a positive step to avoid the bigotry of some secularists. which borders on the totalitarian.[175]

4.3 Public Debate in a Pluralist Society

Every intelligent participant in public debate needs to face the question of how to conduct oneself in pluralist debate and what are legitimate personal ambitions for that participation.

---

[173] Charles Journet, *The Meaning of Grace,* (London: Chapman 1960), p. 117.
[174] John Fleming private communication 24/9/2009.
[175] Ibid.

To expect to produce public policy to one's liking would be an aspiration to demagoguery or tyranny. More than that, it would offend against basic ideals of freedom. It is not unreasonable, however, to expect that public debate on matters of public policy be about achieving a pluralist rationale for public policy and, in that sense, a public morality.

We do not live in isolation but in community. We do need a public morality, a set of values that underlies our public structures and institutions and guides our conduct in community. Some basic norms are required for people to live together harmoniously.

To that end, we each have a personal responsibility to seek to know the truth and to engage in discussion about the moral norms and public policy. Those who take that search for truth seriously, from idealists like Immanuel Kant, libertarians like John Stuart Mill through to religious conservatives, have upheld the view that the pursuit of truth is best served by protecting each person from external coercion, from anything that would impinge upon his or her psychological freedom or would prevent individuals from freely associating or freely expressing their views. The right to freedom of thought, conscience and religion is essential for the protection of many other rights, and ought not to be impeded, provided that just public order is protected.

The search for truth, then, is an inquiry that should be free and informed and developed by dialogue. Freedom of association and free moral discussion are a crucial part of that inquiry.

Society also has the right to defend itself and its citizens against possible abuses committed on the pretext of freedom of religion (eg genital mutilation of women – though that is more a cultural phenomenon than a religious practice). But governments should not be arbitrary or unfair in that respect. Government has responsibilities to safeguard the rights of all citizens and for the peaceful settlement of conflicts of rights. Peace comes about when people live together in ways that respect the dignity and rights of each.

There is a thus need for a public morality, a set of norms that govern our relationships with each other based on the fundamental notion of equal respect for persons, our inherent dignity, and our inalienable rights. These notions constitute the basic components of the common good. Outside of these restraints and obligations of the common good, persons have freedom in full range.

4.4 State Neutrality about Religion in Australia

A legitimate aim of involvement in public debate is to seek to develop policies that give expression to equal respect for persons. There are many differences of opinion as to what constitutes respect for persons and indeed what is meant by "human dignity." That discussion is fruitful and worthwhile, and the contributions of a plurality of approaches deepen and strengthen understanding. Open public debate thus serves important functions.

The point is not to exclude considered perspectives from discussion, but to listen to each and to gain the insights that each brings. Bigotry is limiting and destructive of community precisely because it is an effort to isolate and exclude contributions from discussion. In recent times we have witnessed the extraordinary bigotry of exclusive secularism that has attempted to exclude religious perspectives from public discussion.

As an example of this form of secularist activism, American jurist Ronald Dworkin asserts the essentially *religious* content of respect for the intrinsic value of human life. He argues that State enforcement of responsibilities to protect the intrinsic value of human life would breach the First Amendment and the understanding that a state has no business prescribing what people should think about the ultimate value of human life, about why human life has intrinsic importance, and about how that value is respected or dishonoured in different circumstances.[176]

This argument is linked in Australia to the Australian Constitution. Section 116 provides:

---

[176] Ronald Dworkin, *Life's Dominion*, (New York: Knopf, 1993) p. 164.

The Commonwealth shall not make any law for establishing any religion, or for imposing any religious observance, or for prohibiting the free exercise of any religion, and no religious test shall be required as a qualification for any office or public trust under the Commonwealth.

The meaning of section 116 was determined by the High Court of Australia in the famous "Defence of Government Schools" (DOGS) case in 1981 which Justice Barwick CJ found "...the establishment of religion must be found to be the object of the making of the law. Further, because the whole expression is "for establishing any religion," the law to satisfy the description must have that objective as its express and, as I think, single purpose.[177]

The purpose of these provisions in the Australian Constitution is, then, to limit the role of the State, not to limit the role of the Church or any other religious grouping. Having come from a society where the King nationalised religion and made the Church a department of State under parliamentary control, persecuting and marginalising those whose religious opinions differed from those of the State, it is not surprising that the founders wanted a constitution that would allow maximum freedom of religion. Where religion is concerned, it is the Church that needs protection from the hubris of politicians and not vice versa. The Church did not impose religion upon England. England imposed its views on the Church.[178]

Moreover, the Australian Constitution does not exclude religious arguments, religious people, or the Churches from public debate. The opposite is true. People are not to have their religious freedom infringed by the state and are to be permitted to express their religious opinions in the public square. The Australian Constitution itself recognises the legitimacy of religion in the public square when, in its

---

[177] *Black v. The Commonwealth* (1981) HCA 2, (1981) 146 CLR 559 (2 February 1981), at 579, http://www.austlii.edu.au/au/cases/cth/HCA/1981/2.html.
[178] I am indebted to John Fleming in a chapter we co-authored entitled "Seeking a Consensus" in John Fleming and Nicholas Tonti-Filippini (Eds) *Common Ground? Seeking an Asutralian Consensus on Abortion and Sex Education* St Paul Publications 2007 pp. 312-330.

Preamble, it says that we, the Australian people, are "humbly relying on the blessings of Almighty God." This is further supported by the custom of the Parliament to begin each day with prayer including the "Our Father."[179]

Perhaps it is fairer to say that the Australian Constitution provides for the cooperation between Church and state, religion and state. Michael Hogan, Research Associate in Government and International Relations at The University of Sydney, put it this way:

> Australia does not have a legally entrenched principle, or even a vague set of conventions, of the separation of church and state. From the appointment of Rev. Samuel Marsden as one of the first magistrates in colonial New South Wales, to the adoption of explicit policies of state aid for denominational schools during the 1960s, to the two examples mentioned above, Australia has had a very consistent tradition of cooperation between church and state. "Separation of church and state," along with "the separation of powers" or "pleading the Fifth," are phrases that we have learned from the US, and which merely serve to confuse once they are taken out of the context of the American Constitution.[180]

What Australia does have is a principle of state *neutrality*, or equal treatment, when dealing with churches. This principle dates back at least to Governor Bourke (if not to Macquarie) in colonial NSW, and extends all the way into contemporary Australia where government monies at all levels go quite happily to the churches so that they can run schools, hospitals, employment agencies, social welfare bureaux and even drug injecting rooms. This principle of neutrality is not entrenched in either the State or Federal Constitutions, and has no legal standing. (Constitutionally, State governments could still conceivably nominate an established church; only the Commonwealth is forbidden to do so by Section 116 of its Constitution!) Ultimately, the strength of the principle comes from the conventions hammered out in colonial

---
[179] Ibid.
[180] Ibid.

Australia that saw English and Scottish established churches deprived of their priority in government funding. It survives into the twenty-first century because no major party could seriously contemplate abandoning it.[181]

The principle of state neutrality has coexisted in Australia with a strong secular tradition in politics in the sense that there is no official church and no expectation that what the Church or Churches might say would be translated into law. For most of our history, most Australians have been quite happy with the principle that governments should not favour one church over another.[182]

4.5 Bigotry about Participation of Religion

Notwithstanding the legal position, many politicians and others have behaved in a way that does not respect the Australian Constitution by demanding that bishops, priests, ministers, churches, and other religious bodies stop "meddling" in politics. Such *ad hominem* attacks represent an egregious appeal to prejudice and unjust discrimination against certain people or institutions. It is also hypocritical in the strict sense because such advice is usually given by, but not expected to apply to, those whose religion is variously described as secular, "humanist", atheistic, or agnostic.

Examples of publicly expressed religious bigotry by significant members of the press, political establishment, and others abound. The views of Christians are associated with fundamentalism, that unenlightened and ignorantly dogmatic religion, which is impervious to science, reason, and compassion. Alex Mitchell, columnist for Sydney's *The Sun Herald*, exemplified the crudest expression of anti-Catholic bigotry when accounting for the way in which NSW Senators voted against a private member's bill to overturn the ban on therapeutic cloning in 2006. Senators Ursula Stephens and Steve Hutchins were

---
[181] Ibid.
[182] Michael Hogan, "Separation of Church and State?" 16 May 2001 http://www.australianreview.net/digest/2001/05/hogan.html.

described as coming "from the darkest recesses of the NSW right," while Senators Bill Heffernan and Concetta Fierravanti-Wells were "mediaevalists" who "took their stand somewhere around the fifteenth century when the Spanish Inquisition was in full swing."[183]

Senator Amanda Vanstone, in supporting therapeutic cloning, said, "There are different views on when life begins, but no religion has the right to seek to have its view legislated." Never mind that Senator Vanstone then voted to have her own religious views legislated. Each politician was expected to vote, and Vanstone cast her vote according to her own opinion. But she was wrong to tell politicians of a different religious opinion to her own that they did not have the same right to seek to persuade the Parliament to a particular point of view. There is nothing in the Australian Constitution to justify the denial of equal rights to free speech on the basis of a person's religious or other opinions.

The Hon. Tony Abbott was constantly questioned about his objectivity and even his right to be able to hold the office of Minister for Health because he is a Catholic. This was a constant theme in the debate over the abortion drug RU-486. And the same line of questioning of his religious views continued in relation to the therapeutic cloning debate.

> *Question:* Do you get the feeling that every time you open your mouth on these issues of conscience or ethics people – your critics – impugn your motives because of your religious faith?
>
> *Tony Abbott:* I think that it's noteworthy that no one was demanding that religion be kept out of politics when Bruce Baird, Barnaby Joyce, and Stephen Fielding opposed the Government's immigration bill but, on this particular issue, there are enormous demands, including from prominent members of the Labor Party, that "religion" be kept out of politics.

---

[183] Alex Mitchell, "Faulkner Lone State ALP Senator to Back Cloning Legislation," *The Sun Herald*, November 12, 2006, p. 22.

Now, the truth is that I certainly haven't injected religion into politics, and I don't believe on the stem cell issue or the cloning issue anyone has injected religion into politics. The arguments that I've used, and other opponents of change in this area have used, are all based on human values. They're not based on religious teaching.

Question: But it's a religious issue. Stem cells is a religious issue, and you could easily argue that case as well, couldn't you?

Tony Abbott: Well, I – my arguments are not based on religious teaching. They're not based on Scripture; they're not based on what the Pope or the Archbishop of Canterbury or the Dalai Lama has said – they're based on what I think are decent human values that can be apprehended by anyone, regardless of his or her religious views.[184]

Abbott exemplified the classical Catholic approach to debating moral issues in the public square when he insisted that he was arguing on the basis of agreed "human values" (the wrongfulness of killing the innocent), and the scientific account of when human life begins. He did not appeal to data that are the sole preserve of revelation.

To make it clear that people should discount views contrary to those held by the elites, media outlets commonly describe dissenters as "devout Catholic" or "fundamentalist." We have yet to see anyone from the elites described as "atheist" or "agnostic." Which begs the question, "Why not?" All human beings are influenced by their personal religious and philosophical commitments. Why is this only to be considered a problem for Christians? The attempt to define out of public debate contributors who come from selected religious viewpoints (but not others) exemplifies how deeply anti-religious and sectarian bigotry goes, especially among those who would regard themselves as "enlightened," even "educated."

---

[184] "Doorstop Interview–Herceptin listed on the PBS," August 22, 2006, http://www.health.gov.au/internet/ministers/publishing.nsf/Content/health-mediarel-yr2006-ta-abbsp220806.htm?OpenDocument&yr=2006&mth=8.

4.6 Religious Participation in the Public Square

When people of religious persuasion, either as individuals or in company with others of similar mind, take part in public discussion, they do so legitimately simply as citizens expressing a view about the common good and the principles that are needed to protect the common good. They are behaving responsibly by taking their civic role seriously, provided of course that they conduct themselves properly within the norms of the Australian democratic system. This caveat also applies to those who replace intelligent argument and debate with *ad hominem* attacks that invite people to disregard fellow citizens on the basis of their religion.

A major issue in this respect has been respect for human life. The view that human life is to be protected is implied by the simple idea of equal respect for persons. As such, it is expressed as a right in the international human rights instruments, and in fact the only right that is explicitly recognised in the instruments as an inherent right (ICCPR n. 6). It is legitimate to argue about who is a person, but that is not essentially a religious debate, even if religious people may be inclined to be more sensitive to the need to protect those who are most vulnerable on the fringes of life.

The Australian Constitution protects religious freedom, including freedom of association and of expression. The right to be involved in public debate is therefore protected. It is manifestly unjust and extraordinarily bigoted to claim that religious people ought not to be permitted to contribute or that their contribution ought not to be considered.

At the same time, contribution to public debate needs to be aware of the sensitivities of others. Public policy advances through seeking points of agreement and being careful to respect areas of disagreement. There is a role for what John Rawls[185] calls "public reason." The latter is a discussion that takes place on the basis of agreed fundamental principles.

---

[185] John Rawls, "The Idea of Public Reason Revisited" in John Rawls, *The Law of Peoples* (1999) Harvard University Press, 1999.

However it is important that there is also continued discussion of those fundamental principles, as well as on the application of them, and it is appropriate in a pluralist society that all perspectives are brought to bear upon that discussion in a considered way.

The great traditions in every age and culture have tended to identify the very same core values. Our human need for a transcendent reality that is beyond the merely human ultimately outlasts every other alternative belief form both intellectually and emotionally.

4.7 Secularism and Protecting Religious Freedom

As discussed, a bigoted form of secularism has emerged as a form of belief that is intolerant of religious viewpoints and seeks to exclude them from the formation of public policy. This is to be distinguished from a form of secularism that is genuinely pluralist in that it acknowledges the place of the range of different belief systems, cultures and traditions in the task of developing public policy. Earlier, I described my own experience of that form of secularism in the practical development of public policy.

In contemporary Australia society, the bigoted version of secularism is a threat to a tolerant, democratic society. Because that is so, it has become obvious that the freedom of thought, conscience and religion that have long existed in Australia can no longer be taken for granted. Australian law does not protect freedom of thought, conscience and religion. The discussion of the possibility of a law in relation to religious freedom is thus taking place against a background in which the mood of aggressive secularism is not to protect religious freedom, but rather to curtail it.

It is therefore important to be clear about what kind of society we wish Australia to be, and to understand that both religious fundamentalists and aggressive secularists are opposed to Australia being a tolerant and democratic society in which everyone has a place at the table of public reason.

In a recent address to an Oxford audience, Cardinal George Pell discussed the emergence of pluralist intolerance and the trend toward the law being used to give expression to that intolerance. He gave many contemporary examples in which the law is being used to oppress religion in Western society, including:

- the recent Victorian *Abortion Law Reform Act* 2008, which overrides the right to freedom of thought, conscience and religion by requiring doctors either to provide or at least to refer for abortion, and nurses to provide abortion at a doctor's request;
- the likelihood that President Obama will keep his commitment to sign into law a proposed "Freedom of Choice Act," which will sweep away any restrictions on abortion in state laws and which will also remove any protections in legislation for doctors, nurses, and hospitals with moral objections to abortion;
- the legalisation of same-sex marriage in Canada, which does not allow civil celebrants the right to decline to bless such marriages;
- anti-discrimination laws that raise serious freedom of religion issues for churches in the areas of relationship counselling, sex and relationship education in secondary schools, the hire of parish, school and church facilities, and accommodation arrangements in emergency housing, retreat, conference and aged care centres;
- religious vilification and hate crime legislation, which created the circumstances in which, in separate cases in Canada last year, human rights tribunals brought charges of hate crime against the publisher Ezra Levant (for republishing the cartoons of Muhammad which were first printed in the Danish newspaper *Jyflands-Posten* in 2005) and the weekly magazine *Macleans* (for publishing an excerpt from Mark Steyn's 2006 book *America Alone* under the title "The Future belongs to Islam"). In 2006 Italian journalist Oriana Fallaci was charged with vilifying

Islam in her book *The Force of Reason,* and in 2004 two Australian evangelical pastors were brought before a tribunal in the Australian state of Victoria for critical remarks about Islam which were alleged to be in breach of Victoria's "religious tolerance" legislation.

- "contraceptive mandate" laws, passed in eighteen states of the US, usually with names such as The Women's Contraceptive Equity Act or The Women's Health and Wellness Act, which require employer health insurance plans to cover the costs of contraceptives on the basis that failure to do so constitutes sex discrimination. Catholic health insurance usually did not cover these costs.

The Cardinal writes:

> Modern liberalism has strong totalitarian tendencies. Institutions and associations, it implies, exist only with the permission of the state and to exist lawfully, they must abide by the dictates or norms of the state. Modern liberalism is remote indeed from traditional liberalism, which sees the individual and the family and the association as prior to the state, with the latter existing only to fulfil functions that the former require but which are beyond their means to provide. Traditional liberalism understood the state to exist to assist (provide *subsidium)* to the association; the association does not exist to further the function of the state. All this is clearly articulated in the *Universal Declaration of Human Rights* (1948) which provides, for example, that parents have "a prior right to choose the kind of education that shall be given to their children" (Article 26(3)); and in the *International Covenant on Economic and Social and Cultural Rights* (1966) which provides that the state is to respect the liberty of parents "to ensure the religious and moral education of their children in

conformity with their own convictions" (Article 13(3)).[186]

Secular intolerance and bigotry should be seen in the same way as religious intolerance and religious fundamentalism: both have the capacity for harm by seeking to exclude others. The anti-democratic nature of bigoted secularism needs to be recognised, in its seeking to dominate the formation of public policy and development of law on the basis that it alone has the exclusive right to be heard in the public domain. Secularism is not a neutral view. It is a view based on beliefs that exclude belief in a Deity. As such, it can claim a right to be heard in a democracy, but no greater right than any other view. It also merits criticism for its bigotry.

The inclusion of the range of views within pluralism is particularly important in relation to developing inter-faith harmony and co-operation for the social and economic well-being of Australia and safeguarding it from extremism of all kinds. The latter goal is one of the major recommendations of the Report *Religion, Cultural Diversity and Safeguarding Australia*[187] prepared on behalf of the Department of Immigration and Multicultural and Indigenous Affairs and the Australian Multicultural Foundation in association with the World Conference of Religions for Peace, RMIT University and Monash University.

If secularist views, as opposed to religious views, are able to lay claim to an exclusive right to be heard, then those who have religious beliefs have reason to be fearful. In this context, there is scepticism about the goals of the Australian Human Rights Commission *Freedom of Religion and Belief in the 21st Century* project because the project takes place against a background of aggressive and very bigoted secularism. The response of the Victorian Ad Hoc Interfaith Committee to the discussion paper on the project typifies religious concern about

---

[186] Cardinal George Pell, "Varieties of Intolerance: Religious and Secular" Inaugural Hilary Term Lecture, Oxford University Newman Society, The Divinity School, Oxford University, 9 March 2009 http://www.scribd.com/doc/13065181/Varieties-of-Intolerance-Religious-and-Secular-George-Cardinal-Pell.
[187] http://amf.net.au/library/file/Religion_Cultural_Diversity_Main_Report.pdf Accessed 24/9/09.

its merits:

The question, Q 5.8, page 8 of the Discussion Paper, "is there a role for religious voices alongside others in the policy debates of the nation?" is a strange question given ICCPR, Article 25.

The presence of this question as well as questions Qs 2.3 and 2.4, page 9 when coupled with Mr Calma's reputed comments[188] made at the launch of FRB Project: *("Does religious belief influence policies being determined in any country, particularly in our country?" he said. Mr Calma says there is a balance to be struck between the freedom to practice a religion and not pushing those beliefs on the rest of society.")* brings the question to our minds as to whether the FRB Project is in fact predicated on the assumption that secularism is the proper default position for public discourse and that the project is not about freedom *of* religion, but rather freedom *from* religion. We are well aware that many secularists hold this opinion. It would be particularly unfortunate and certainly would undermine the credibility of the FRB Review if this was the case for this project.[189]

An important element of the project should be to recognise the legitimate place in the development of public policy of those who give expression to religious beliefs. No-one in a democracy should be made to feel that public policy belongs to any particular belief system, other than belief in the nature of democracy to serve every member of the community and to represent every member of the community. It is an important feature of political victory speeches in Australia that the leader of the victorious party claims to serve not just those who elected them, but every member of the community. Protecting the

---

[188] ABC Radio (http://www.abc.net.au/news/stories/2008/09/17/2366511.htm?section=justin) report of the launch of the FRB project.

[189] Submission 1687 from the Victorian Ad Hoc Interfaith Committee to the Australian Human Rights Commission *Freedom of Religion and Belief in the 21st Century* Project http://www.hreoc.gov.au/frb/frb_submissions.html (Note that the author is a joint chairperson of the Ad Hoc Interfaith Committee and a signatory to submission 1687).

openness and fairness of Australian society means not allowing any particular group to lay claim to an exclusive role in the formation of public policy and law.

The development of a law to protect religious freedom needs to have as its premise the equality before such a law of each person, no matter the beliefs that he or she may hold. It is his or her right to express those beliefs in the public forum as a contribution to public discussion, and no form of belief is to be given a superior role in the process of developing public policy.

Given that religious belief is the subject of a proposed law to protect religious freedom, it is important also that each belief system be permitted to define its own beliefs and practices and their priority within that belief system. That would seem to be part of what is meant by religious freedom.

The tension that is likely to arise in the development of a religious freedom law is in the potential for conflict between, on the one hand, religious beliefs and practices within religious institutions and their agencies, and, on the other, the norms of conduct adopted by the wider society. This is evident, for instance, in the tension over applying principles of non-discrimination, so appropriate in the conduct of wider society, to a religious institution, which seeks to give witness to particular beliefs and thus to allocate educative or leadership roles to those who give practical expression to those beliefs, including moral beliefs about lifestyle; or which limits roles in ministry on the basis of beliefs about gender.

The issue in those circumstances is whether beliefs and practices within the institution or its agency may be overridden by norms of conduct that are proper to the wider society. There would seem to be a difference between making and implementing policy and law for wider society and applying those policies and laws to the internal conduct of religion. Many of the fears expressed about the development of a law to protect religious freedom are based on the possibility that the law will be used to override religious beliefs and practices.

Distinctions need to be made between harmful practices that might be carried out in the name of religious belief or culture, such as genital mutilation, (though there is little evidence that this practice is based on religious belief – it appears to be more a cultural tradition), and practices that do not cause harm, for example, limiting the role of a minister of religion according to gender, based on belief, or the practice of employing people in educative or leadership roles on the basis of their giving practical witness to the beliefs and practices of the religion. Those seeking to develop a law to protect religious freedom will need to articulate some distinctions between what might properly be regarded as being defined by religious belief and beyond the scope of the law to determine, and those matters in which the law overrides religious belief and practice in order to protect other important rights, such as the right to bodily integrity or the right to freedom of association.

A tension that has emerged in this respect is the conflict between freedom of thought, conscience and religion on the one hand and legislation that requires health professionals to provide services that may be contrary to their conscientiously held moral beliefs. Those framing legislation to protect religious freedom will need to make a decision about the effect of the law with respect to conscientious objection, whether it does or does not protect it.

5

Public Reason and the Case of Bioethics[190]

5.1 A Catholic in a Pluralist Environment

This chapter is offered as a personal experience of the openness of Australian society to religious contribution in public policy formation. To that extent, it describes what may be considered something of an ideal of pluralist public policy formation.

For many years I have practised as a consultant bioethicist and in that role have served Australian governments, both State and Federal, and on government committees. I have also served as a consultant to the Office of Technology Assessment of the US Congress and to the German Federal Department of Health and Welfare.

Though holding secular qualifications in Philosophy, I have never made a secret of my status as a practicing Catholic. From time to time I have drawn criticism for that, no more so than when in 2006 I was a member of an Australian Health Ethics Committee (AHEC) subcommittee on reproductive technology and a submission from a major university to the committee attacked my membership on the grounds of my religious beliefs. (AHEC is a principal committee of the National Health and Medical Research Council – the NHMRC.)

---

[190] A large part of this section is drawn from an article entitled "Public Reason and Bioethics," which has been accepted for publication in the journal *New Blackfriars*.

As a general rule, my involvement in public policy development has been tolerated, although in the public forum, rather than being classified just in terms of my profession, the media generally insist on mentioning that I am Catholic, though they do not as a rule mention the religious beliefs of other participants in debate. This to some extent indicates secularist bigotry, as though readers, listeners or viewers need to be warned that the view that they are about to hear is a Catholic view, but other types of view need no such warning.

The circumstance referred to above in which I was criticised by a major university and thus a major client of the NHMRC for my beliefs, thankfully did not require me to offer a defence of my role on the committee in the process of developing public policy as a person with religious convictions. The submission had asserted that I should be excluded from membership of the committee. The NHMRC did not ask me to resign and, sensibly in my view, did not respond to, act on or make public the comments that referred to me in that way. Had they done so in a way that was to my disadvantage, however, there would seem to be nothing in Australian law that would have protected me against discrimination on the basis of my beliefs, though an argument might have been put on the basis of a section 116 of the Constitution, and also that the Australian Government as a signatory to the International Covenant on Civil and Political Rights had an obligation to protect me under clause 18.

Given that protection of freedom of religion is the subject of this present discussion, it is useful to explain, first, the right of a person with religious convictions to be involved in the development of public policy. This explanation reflects a view about the way a tolerant pluralist society should operate in relation to allowing participation in public policy formation.

Central to Christian ethics is a concept of human dignity founded on the *imago Dei*, and informed by the life and teachings of Jesus Christ. The Church however has many voices: prophetic, academic/

professional, humanistic and artistic.[191] In the field of bioethics, the proclamation of the Word of God and witness to the person and teachings of Christ are prophetic and essential, from a Christian perspective, but not always the voice that a pluralist audience is prepared to hear. More importantly, out of respect for the differing beliefs of others, one would not attempt to speak prophetically where there is no shared basis of belief.

Bioethics, as a pluralist system of regulation of biomedical research and practice, demands a voice other than the prophetic. For a Christian, upholding the dignity of the human person within Bioethics calls us to develop a language and reasoning that belongs to the pluralist rather than the religious world. This of course may be seen by some as a conflict with the vocation of a Christian. It also means buying into the debate represented by the comment of the then Cardinal Ratzinger (now Pope Benedict XVI) that "reason has a wax nose," by which he meant that the shape of reason is determined by theological convictions.[192] In his 1996 address to the Congregation of the Doctrine of the Faith, "Current Situation of Faith and Theology," Cardinal Ratzinger agreed with Karl Barth's rejection of philosophy as the foundation of faith independent of faith, but rejected Barth's claim that faith is a pure paradox that can only exist against reason and totally independent from it. He called for a new dialogue between faith and philosophy. "Reason," he said, "will not be saved without the faith, but the faith without reason will not be human."[193]

My own understanding of the role of philosophy reflects the late Pope John Paul II's comment:

> Every people has its own native and seminal wisdom which, as
> a true cultural treasure, tends to find voice and develop in forms

---

[191] John W. O'Malley, *Four Cultures of the West*, (London: Harvard University Press, 2004), p. 7.
[192] Tracey Rowland, *Ratzinger's Faith: The Theology of Pope Benedict XVI, (Oxford:* OUP, 2008) p. 5.
[193] Cardinal Joseph Ratzinger, An address to the Congregation of the Doctrine of the Faith, "Current Situation of Faith and Theology" 1996 http://www.ourladyswarriors. org/dissent/ratzsitu596.htm (Accessed June 18, 2008).

which are genuinely philosophical. One example of this is the basic form of philosophical knowledge which is evident to this day in the postulates which inspire national and international legal systems in regulating the life of society.[194]

The task of a national bioethics committee, such as the one on which I served for some years, is to seek to be a part of the project of developing and applying those values that can be truly considered a "cultural treasure." In that respect I hope to have given expression to the concluding words to philosophers of Pope John Paul II in his letter "Faith and Reason":

> They should be open to the impelling questions which arise from the word of God and they should be strong enough to shape their thought and discussion in response to that challenge. Let them always strive for truth, alert to the good which truth contains. Then they will be able to formulate the genuine ethics which humanity needs so urgently at this particular time. The Church follows the work of philosophers with interest and appreciation; and they should rest assured of her respect for the rightful autonomy of their discipline. I would want especially to encourage believers working in the philosophical field to illumine the range of human activity by the exercise of a reason which grows more penetrating and assured because of the support it receives from faith.

I do not see that there is a dichotomy between faith and reason, or between theology and philosophy. Philosophy would be foolish indeed if it willingly blinded itself to theology and to Scripture and resolved never to consider propositions that emerge from consideration of the nature of the Creator and the relationship between created and Creator. What is different about philosophy is that it resolves to test those propositions against reason and to seek justification, rather than accept them simply as a matter of faith. For a Christian, there is no difficulty in believing the teachings of Christ to be true, and, because they are

---

[194] *Fides et Ratio*, n. 4.

true, considering them able to withstand the examination of reason.

It would be mistaken to think that, because in a pluralist society we cannot expect that others share our faith, we must not introduce Christian notions, and if we do, they must be under some other guise. Such subterfuge is beneath dignity. It is better to go into a committee meeting or a Parliament known for one's faith in Christ Jesus, but also for one's willingness to listen to others and to explore concepts with a view to seeking truth that is broadly recognisable by others. In other words, one seeks, as a matter of mutual respect, common ground between one's own unashamed and obviously Christian beliefs and the beliefs of others, and with a willingness to question and to explore together what is true and good.

In his earlier critique of the Vatican document *Gaudium et Spes*, Ratzinger asserts that:

> ... it seemed to many people, especially from German speaking countries, that there was not a radical enough rejection of a doctrine of man divided into philosophy and theology. They were convinced that fundamentally the text was still based on a schematic representation of nature and the supernatural viewed far too much as merely juxtaposed. To their mind it took as its starting point the fiction that it is possible to construct a rational philosophical picture of man intelligible to all and on which all men of goodwill can agree, the actual Christian doctrines being added to this as a sort of crowning conclusion.[195]

He goes on to attribute this error to the Thomists:[196] "It can hardly be disputed that as a consequence of the division between philosophy and theology established by the Thomists, a juxtaposition has gradually been established which no longer appears adequate. There is, and must

---

[195] Joseph Ratzinger, "The Dignity of the Human Person" in Herbert Vorgrimler (ed) *Commentary on the Documents of Vatican II* Volume V, (London: Burns & Oates, 1969), pp. 115-163.

[196] Those who follow in the philosophical tradition of St. Thomas Aquinas who is A Middle Ages philosopher/theologian who applied the writing of the Ancient Greek philosopher Aristotle to the task of natural theology.

be, a human reason *in* faith, yet conversely, every human reason is conditioned by historical standpoint so that reason pure and simple does not exist."[197]

It is worth noting in this respect Ratzinger's emphasis on historical standpoint, and thus on culture and tradition, is also a basis for much of the philosopher Alasdair MacIntyre's approach, and the latter has drawn criticism on the grounds of relativism for it.

My own experience in working within a pluralist environment towards an agreed policy on matters of public ethics is that each of us does bring our own culture and tradition and that is likely to include theological traditions. What is spoken about, however, is not theology as such, but rather the search for a set of agreed and basic values upon which a coherent policy can be formulated. The reasons why we each uphold a basic value is not so much discussed as accepted, and what then emerges is a position that both is determined by individual culture, and also which transcends individual culture because it is held in common across cultures and has been subjected to scrutiny and the need for justification on its own propositional terms.

A philosopher thus has more to contribute to that discussion than a theologian, precisely because as philosophers we are interested in exploring why a teaching is good for mankind and justifying it in human terms. A Christian philosopher regards him or herself as informed by faith but willing to see philosophical propositions tested for their justification, believing that what God wants for us is good for us because he loves us.

My response to the claim that reason will not be saved without faith is that independent of faith, goodness is a property that is recognizable by those who are unfamiliar with the Scriptures. In public discussion involving people who belong to a range of faiths and none, it is legitimate and worthwhile to work together to find a common understanding of human goodness and what we call the Pauline Principle – never do evil (that is, act against human goodness) to achieve good. Faith is informative and not separate from our experience of the good, but the

---

[197] Ibid.

good also appears to be a property that remains recognisable by those of no apparent faith. Faiths are not to be excluded from that pursuit, for that would be both arrogant and bigoted, but the task is one of seeking to find that which is transcendent of individual faith, culture and tradition.

In discussing virtue, St Thomas Aquinas accepted the division of virtues and saw the cardinal virtues (wisdom, justice, restraint and courage) as distinct from the religious virtues (faith, hope and love), holding that all virtues other than the religious or theological are in us by nature, according to aptitude and inchoation, but not according to perfection. The theological virtues, he claims, are from without.[198] By that he means that the cardinal virtues belong to reason alone and recognised simply by reflecting on our human experience, but the theological virtues do require a source external to us, namely revelation of divine truth in the person and teaching of Christ, for them to attain their deepest and fullest meaning.

From practical experience in consulting in ethics within the practice of psychiatry, I would claim that the cardinal virtues transcend tradition and culture simply because to lack any one of them completely would be a form of mental illness. One only has to consider what it would be like to be totally without wisdom and thus unable to identify goodness, or to be totally without courage and thus unable to venture out, or to be totally without justice and thus lack a sense of the needs of others, or totally without restraint and thus be unable to control one's passions or inclinations. The cardinal virtues are essential to living in community.

The religious virtues, however, presuppose a God, but they are not without philosophical justification independent of faith in the person of Christ, who so illuminates them by his personal witness and teaching. They belong to all religious traditions, not just Christianity.

People who believe in a divinity are entitled to seek to understand

---

[198] "Sic ergo patet quod virtutes in nobis sunt a natura secundum aptitudinem et inchoationem, non autem secundum perfectionem: prater virtutes theologicas, quae sunt totaliter ab extrinseco"S. Thomae Aquinatis *Summa Theologiae* (Marietti: Taurini/ Romae 1952) Prima Secundae Partis Q. 63, Articulus I.

human nature through theological sources, and they are entitled to offer the fruits of their researchers to the wider community to be evaluated for merit and worth. I would argue from the basis of a Christian understanding that human beings are designed for communion, that true human happiness and human fulfilment only ever occur as a result of gift of self, and that that understanding does provide a depth of meaning for marriage and human sexuality. In this respect I hold that John Paul II did not replace appeal to what is supposedly "against nature" with a radically biblical doctrine of the spousal relationship (or nuptiality), as some have claimed,[199] but rather he has insisted on understanding sexuality in terms of the communion of persons that is our ultimate vocation and which finds expression in this life in the gifts of marriage and, by analogy, committed celibacy.

In other words far from decrying the "against nature" arguments, Pope John Paul II has instead developed the notion of what is a human nature, with part of that nature being the vocation toward forming a communion of persons. For a Christian the *imago Dei* is not of a single person but of a communion of three persons. The relationship of each to the other thus provides the goal and the model for human relationships.

The task for Christian philosophy is the task that the late Pope John Paul II gave himself in his doctoral dissertation, *The Acting Person*, of understanding human nature in a vocationally relational way. This is far from rendering non-theological ethics redundant. It is important that these developments of an understanding of human nature are challenged and justified on philosophical terms. It is only by doing so that the Scriptural understanding of the human person, which is the basis of the John Paul II's Wednesday audiences on *Theology of the Body*, for instance, can gain credibility through its internal coherence and consistency in philosophical terms.

When we are able to do that, we will then have a conceptual framework that can be used in the engagement with our society. The

---

[199] See for instance, Fergus Kerr *Twentieth Century Catholic Theologians*, (Oxford: Blackwell, 2007), p. 179.

greatest distance between Christian moral understanding and our Western culture occurs at the level of understanding of the spousal relationship. There is an urgent need to try to bridge that gap with a philosophical analysis of human nature that gives substance and justification to giving oneself in love. We need a way of constructing a common ground with others.

Critical analysis and evaluation as I was taught it at as a Philosophy post-graduate was a process that one learned, by which the worth of a philosophical work could be judged by the number of distinctions made and defended. This approach has had its detractors. The philosopher Alasdair MacIntyre argues that contemporary philosophy has condemned itself to engaging in irresolvable or, more precisely, stagnating disputes by virtually making a virtue out of difference and of splintering of positions. He claims:

> Modern academic philosophy turns out by and large to provide means for a more accurate and informed definition of disagreement rather than for progress toward its resolution. Professors of philosophy who concern themselves with questions of justice and of practical rationality turn out to disagree with each other as sharply, as variously and, so it seems, as irremediably upon how such questions are to be answered as anyone else.[200]

In my own experience on ethics committees and shaping policy, the much more important matter is not the fine points of disagreement and difference, but the development of agreement and consensus, for it is upon the latter that policy actually develops. In my own teaching I have come to recognize that an important skill for Bioethics graduates to learn is how to analyse and evaluate toward a resolution, not to achieve more difference.

I have found that good graduate student essays have picked up the need to consider a range of views, and to work with the different concepts within those differences. Their method, however, often seems to be little more than to work to a favoured conclusion by dismissing

---

[200] Alasdair MacIntyre, *Whose Justice, Which Rationality,* (London: Duckworth, 1988) p. 3

other views on the basis of identifying some or multiple errors in those positions. Bad student essays did not even get that far and tended to resemble sermons rather than analysis.

The skill, if it can be called that, learned by the students who produced the good essays will be of little use in policy-making or in any public policy forum. Instead of seeking resolution, they have learned to identify difference and then to adopt a view, like supporting a football team, and to support that view by decrying other views through seeking to identify error. Such an approach works against the idea of an ethics committee or policy-making as a process by which advice can be developed that is persuasive and broadly acceptable. The skill that the students acquired was more suited to tyrants and dictators than to a rational democracy.

The much more difficult skill that I think is not well taught is how to use the understanding of difference to work towards consensus. The reality of ethical discussion between people who have different higher order beliefs is that they develop neuralgia points at which their basic higher order beliefs or assumptions are challenged. The skill of seeking resolution is to find words that either avoid or are at least acceptable to the variety of higher order beliefs or assumptions. In that way one can indeed reach a consensus that can be supported from a variety of points of view. An active process of analysis can yield a constructive outcome through the knowledge that that analysis brings. The problem in the student essays discussed above is that they more or less stopped at identifying difference and error, rather than moving on to seek solutions that were constructive.

This might be seen as condoning relativism, a charge that has been levelled at Alasdair MacIntyre, who also holds to respecting a person's culture and tradition. I would counter that the task of an ethics committee is a very practical one of identifying goodness, and goodness is not the preserve of any one culture or tradition, but transcends differences between culture, tradition and religion.

I believe that goodness is indeed real and knowable. The alternative view, that goodness is neither real nor knowable, supports an approach to ethics and public policy that declares the subjectivity and relativity of goodness and that the latter is no more than a positive attitude or liking. For subjectivist views of this nature, public policy seeks only to preserve individual choice. It seeks to avoid making judgements about what is good for human beings and instead treats autonomy as a moral trump. If such an approach dominated, then ethics guidelines would be little more than guidelines for providing information, obtaining consent and appointing representatives for those who lack the capacity. But that is not my experience on government committees and in pluralist bioethics: the function of an ethics committee at both institutional and higher levels is to make a decision about whether a proposal really is good for people and to avoid doing harm to individuals. The real work of an ethics committee depends on identifying what is good for people and what is harmful.

In the task of developing ethical guidelines, it is interesting that pluralist bioethics has had to call on notions that approximate to the Christian concepts of dignity and the language of moral imperatives. A moral language has developed to express ideas such as intrinsic evil and the Pauline principle (never do evil in order to achieve good), and, in Australia at least, there is an as yet unarticulated move away from both autonomy as a moral trump and utilitarian concepts, and towards a theory of the good. This is most clearly expressed in the various ethical guidelines issued by the National Health and Medical Research Council, for which I will give account.

The 1970s and 1980s ideas of replacing utilitarianism with principlism,[201] and principalism's emphasis on autonomy as a moral trump, have given way to ideas of professional integrity and a taxonomy of acts never to be undertaken. It also involves accepting a notion of virtue – the characteristics of a *good* researcher or a *good* clinician. Thus the trend is toward both being influenced by virtue

---

[201] See for instance the approach taken by T L Beauchamp and J F Childress in successive editions of their *Principles of Biomedical Ethics* (2001), though the later editions have tended to move away from autonomy as the dominant value toward a virtue approach.

ethics and adopting a thick notion of the human person and the good of the human person. The teleology that one finds in Christianity, based on seeking communion with God, is not part of a pluralist dialogue, but to some extent the dialogue is still pervaded by an implicit sense of the transcendent nature of humanity.

The history of the dominant view in pluralist Bioethics over the past thirty years can, in large part, be traced through the changing editions of the seminal text of Thomas L Beauchamp and James F. Childress, *Principles of Biomedical Ethics*. Their effort has been to try to capture not the foundations of Bioethics, because there are many and varied approaches that people may take, but what they think is something of a consensus about the principles to be applied on the basis of the variety of approaches. In doing so, they have moved from their early adoption of the principlism of the Belmont Report,[202] the so-called "Georgetown Mantra", and an emphasis on autonomy as the dominant principle. In this shift, they also developed a discomfort with discussing the principle of justice in exclusively utilitarian terms, and then, in the latest edition, they adopted a version of virtue ethics (though lacking a metaphysics or an anthropology, both of which classically inform virtue ethics).

Like other approaches, Christianity in its various forms can contribute to efforts of that nature to help find, at a practical level, a degree of congruence in the application of principles. There are tensions in the way the principles are applied and often a degree of deliberately constructed ambiguity in order to preserve consensus. The important feature, though, is the willingness to seek agreement and to find solutions that are respectful of the different foundational approaches that people from different cultures and traditions may have adopted.

This experience in pluralist bioethics regulation raises some pertinent practical questions about natural law reasoning and the

---

[202] *The Belmont Report, Ethical Principles and Guidelines for the Protection of Human Subjects of Research* The National Commission for the Protection of Human Subjects of Biomedical and Behavioral Research, April 18, 1979.

internal debates within religion about moral epistemology and whether human goods and the moral law are knowable or deducible in a sufficiently rich way as to give rise to an adequate ethic not based on the Word of God.

For me, though, the experience indicated that there is a role for people both with, and without, religious belief in seeking to understand and promote what is good for human beings. Importantly, people of religious beliefs have no less a role in the formation of public policy than anyone else and, in such policy formation, they are entitled to have their ideas heard, whether based on religious belief or not. Those who claim otherwise, I would argue, are both bigoted and undemocratic. Perhaps more importantly, by excluding religious culture they would not only disenfranchise many, they would also be excluding a rich source of ideas about human nature and living in community, and would be abandoning our culture, history, tradition and experience.

This process of seeking agreement across different religious and cultural belief systems is not new or restricted to the NHMRC. It is exactly what was attempted in the development of the international human rights instruments. The Catholic philosopher Jacque Maritain addressed the same question when he asked: "How much agreement can we reach regarding practices even while remaining incurably divided regarding the underlying theory for such practices?"[203] That question was answered in a very practical way by the rich content of the international instruments to which Maritain was a significant contributor and guide, especially the *Universal Declaration on Human Rights* and the two covenants that were its expression in international law: the *International Covenant on Civil and Political Rights* and the *International Covenant on Economic, Social and Cultural Rights*. They were documents to which many different nations, and hence people of many different cultures and religious beliefs, were able to become signatories.

---

[203] M Novak. "Human dignity, human rights" *First Things,* 97 (November) 1999 pp. 39-42.

5.2 The NHMRC Experience[204]

The statutory functions of the Australian Health Ethics Committee (AHEC), a principal committee of the National Health and Medical Research Council (NHMRC), include providing advice or national guidelines about ethical issues in human research and in health care. In fulfilling those tasks, the members of AHEC have been conscious that there is often debate about ethics.

AHEC has noted that ethics is sometimes said to be merely a matter of individual preference or cultural convention. Its response is that although ethical judgments may indeed express personal preferences, and may be connected in complicated ways with cultural conventions, AHEC regards ethics as a form of rational inquiry that concerns how we should live and what we should do.[205]

Further, AHEC has noted that even the best way of reasoning about ethical issues is a matter of debate. For example, some people emphasise the moral undesirability of certain acts (such as deliberate deception) in and of themselves and the moral desirability of certain standards of conduct (such as integrity in one's relationships with others) in and of themselves. Others emphasise the moral significance of anticipating the likely consequences of proposed acts (for example, the likely consequences for a woman who gestates a child for another woman).[206]

Similarly, some people emphasise the duties we owe to each other (for example, the duty to respect another's personal autonomy). Others emphasise the moral claims we are entitled to make against each other (for example, a child's moral entitlement to knowledge of his or her genetic parents).

AHEC holds that all of these kinds of considerations matter, even if there can be reasonable disagreement about how they are

---

[204] I sought and obtained approval from the Chairman of the Australian Health Ethics Committee (AHEC) to use this account of the processes of the NHMRC and the AHEC.
[205] National Health and Medical Research Council, *National Statement on Ethical Conduct in Human Research* Australian Government Canberra 2007 pp. 11-13
[206] Ibid.

to be balanced. In other words, AHEC does not seek to exclude contributions from the various views, but seeks answers to ethical questions based on considering responses from all perspectives. To some extent, that approach is required by the NHMRC Act by which AHEC is established.[207]

The NHMRC Act stipulates the diverse composition of AHEC and the necessity for public consultation in the development of guidelines, and the High Court, no less, has determined, in a case involving the tobacco industry, that not only must there be public consultation, but that the NHMRC must give due regard to what is said in the public consultation submissions. AHEC therefore understands that it is the will of the Parliament that AHEC seeks to prepare advice and guidelines that reflect and to some extent define the values of the Australian community.

Accordingly, in developing ethical guidelines it is necessary for AHEC to ask what are the values at stake and what function do those values have in establishing an ethical basis for practice in research, in clinical practice and in the adoption of public health strategies.

A likely answer may be that we wish to preserve what Australians consider essential for the kind of life they (and their children and grand-children perhaps) wish to live as members of a community. Those values should be reflected in the way that medical research and practice develops, and in the formulation and implementation of public health strategies.

The values and principles of conduct in each context differ because the relationships between people and the responsibilities differ. What is expected of a medical clinician may be different from what is expected of a medical researcher and different again from what may be expected of a manufacturer of therapeutic products or of a government department or agency implementing public health strategies.

---

[207] Ibid.

5.3 AHEC's Values in Research

The *National Statement on Ethical Conduct in Human Research* (NHMRC 2007) describes the relationship between researchers and research participants as the ground on which human research is conducted. The *National Statement* identifies the values of respect for human beings, research merit and integrity, justice, and beneficence as helping to shape that relationship as one of trust, mutual responsibility and ethical equality.

The *National Statement* also acknowledges that while these values have a long history, there are other values that could inform human research, such as altruism, contributing to societal or community goals, and respect for cultural diversity, along with the values that inform *Values and Ethics: Guidelines for Ethical Conduct in Aboriginal and Torres Strait Islander Health Research* (NHMRC 2003): spirit and integrity, reciprocity, respect, equality, survival and protection, and responsibility.

The major value in the *National Statement* is respect for human beings, which is a recognition of each individual's equal intrinsic worth or value. According to AHEC, respect also requires having due regard for the welfare, beliefs, perceptions, customs and cultural heritage, both individual and collective, of those involved in research. It is significant that such a notion of respect for human beings and their intrinsic value is taken as the priority in developing ethical guidelines; as articulated in the *National Statement*, the concept is far removed from the statements of autonomy and individualism that characterize much of the popular pluralist debate.

AHEC goes on to claim that researchers and their institutions should respect the privacy, confidentiality and cultural sensitivities of research participants and, where relevant, of their communities. Any specific agreements made with the participants or the community should be fulfilled.

The *National Statement* also doffs its cap to autonomy in asserting that respect for human beings involves giving due scope, throughout the research process, to the capacity of human beings to make their own decisions. Where participants are unable to make their own decisions or have diminished capacity to do so, respect for them involves empowering them where possible and providing for their protection as necessary. Respect for autonomy has its place, but for the AHEC that produced the *National Statement*, it does not trump respect for the equal individual worth of each member of the human family and judgements about what is good for them.

Whether that remains the case in the future will obviously depend upon the nature of future appointments to AHEC, which is in the hands of the government of the day. However the statutory requirements for the composition of AHEC and for public consultation do presuppose an approach to ethics that is inclusive of, or at least open to, the range of cultures and traditions to be found in Australian society. AHEC should not ever become captive of a particular view and especially not one that is bigoted and exclusive, be it secular or religious. If it did, it would no longer meet the statutory requirements. It is a matter of historical record that the present statutory representative nature of AHEC and the requirements in relation to public consultation arose out of reaction to previous incarnations of the national research ethics body, which did become captive to bigoted and aggressive secularism.

5.4 AHEC's Values in Organ and Tissue Transplantation

In Australia, the donation of organs and tissues after death for transplantation relies on the values of altruism and solidarity, and these values have formed the basis of a system of obtaining and using organs and tissue for transplantation. AHEC has recognized that the medical benefits of this approach to organ and tissue donation have provided a strong motivation for such a system and it is now part of Australia's social capital.

The NHMRC[208] has held that organs and tissues for transplantation after death should be obtained in ways that:

- demonstrate respect for all aspects of human dignity, including the worth, welfare, rights, beliefs, perceptions, customs and cultural heritage of all involved;
- respect the wishes, where known, of the deceased;
- give precedence to the needs of the potential donor and the family over the interests of organ procurement;
- as far as possible, protect recipients from harm; and
- recognise the needs of all those directly involved, including the donor, recipient, families, carers, friends and health professionals.

In the context of a system based on altruism and solidarity, it has been possible to have a process of allocation according to just and transparent processes.

The ethical issues in the donation of living organ and tissue donation principally involve concern for the donors: the autonomy and welfare of the donor take precedence over the needs of the recipient to receive an organ or tissue. The systems in Australia, whether for the blood service, the bone marrow service, the eye bank or solid organ transplantation, have, like those in place for donation after death, been based on altruism and solidarity and respect for human dignity, including the worth of the person and respect for his or her wishes.

5.5 AHEC and Care of People who are Severely Brain Damaged

In 2008, the NHMRC released new ethical guidelines for the care of people in post-coma unresponsiveness (vegetative state) or a minimally

---

[208] National Health and Medical Research Council, *Organ and Tissue Donation by Living Donors: Guidelines for Ethical Practice for health Professionals* Endorsed 15 March 2007; *Organ and Tissue Donation after Death, for Transplantation: Guideliens for Ethical Practice by health Professionals*, Endorsed 15 March 2007.

responsive state.[209] In reference to the vexed issue of withdrawing nutrition and hydration, the guidelines state:

> A person in PCU or MRS may be affected by other conditions, or his or her condition may deteriorate. Complications may also develop in relation to delivering some elements of maintenance care. For example, tube feeding may cause aspiration and recurrent respiratory infection; or a percutaneous endoscopic gastrostomy tube (PEG) may cause excoriation or gut inflammation. People who are minimally responsive may show signs of discomfort.
>
> **The presumption ought to be in favour of continuing maintenance care.** However, such complications may lead to some aspects of maintenance care being considered overly burdensome and they may be withdrawn after careful consultation and informing those involved about the reasons for withdrawal. The person's previously expressed wishes are relevant to a judgement of the burdensomeness of a treatment, and should be considered.
>
> As with any decisions about the treatment of highly dependent patients, **decisions about withholding or withdrawing treatment and the continuing provision of artificial nutrition and hydration should be informed by a consideration of the person's best interests including what, if anything, is known about their wishes; and it should reflect the best contemporary standards of care for people who are highly dependent.** The question is never whether the patient's life is worthwhile, but whether a treatment is worthwhile.

Like all of the recent AHEC documents, these guidelines begin with a statement of ethical principles, which in this document contains the following:

> The provision of care is an expression of our fundamental

---

[209] National Health and Medical Research Council, *Ethical Guidelines for the Care of People in Post Coma Unresponsiveness (Vegetative State) or a Minimally Responsive State*, Australian Government Canberra 2008 http://www.nhmrc.gov.au/publications/synopses/e81_82syn.htm.

humanity and connectedness, and our common sense of obligation to promote good and do no harm. Because of their total dependence on others, people in PCU or MRS are highly vulnerable and, as such, are owed a particular duty of care to promote their interests and protect them from exploitation, abuse and neglect. That duty is likely to extend over a long period of time. Decisions about the care of people in PCU or MRS should:

(a) demonstrate respect for all aspects of human dignity, including the worth, welfare, rights, beliefs, perceptions, customs and cultural heritage of all involved;

(b) respect, where these are known, the values, beliefs and previous wishes of the person in PCU or MRS;

(c) recognise the needs of all those directly involved – including people in PCU or MRS, families, friends, health professionals, and other carers – to be:

   (i) involved in decisions that affect them;

   (ii) given accurate and timely information;

   (iii) realistically educated about the person's situation, care and prospect; and

   (iv) assisted, when necessary, to deal with their own responses in their particular situations;

(d) give due regard to justice, particularly in relation to the responsible use of resources. This includes ensuring so far as possible that there is:

   (i) fair distribution of the benefits of or access to goods and services;

   (ii) equality of opportunity;

   (iii) no unfair burden on any members of the community or on particular groups; and

   (iv) no abuse, neglect, exploitation or discrimination;

(e) respect the basic rights of people in PCU or MRS, including:

   (i) the right of individuals to be treated with respect;

(ii) the right of individuals to life, liberty, and security;
(iii) the right of individuals to have their religious and cultural identity respected;
(iv) the right of competent individuals to self-determination;
(v) the right to a standard of care related to individual needs;
(vi) the right of individuals to privacy and confidentiality;
(vii) the recognition that human beings are social beings with social needs;
(f) give due regard to the rights and duties of those who care for people in PCU and MRS, and the duties of the community both to people in PCU or MRS, and to their carers (family, professional and other);
(g) respect the goals and the limits of medical treatment."

5.6 AHEC's Moral Language

In developing national guidelines for ethical conduct in medical practice and research, AHEC has had to develop a policy about moral language. In the vagaries of committee process, a policy decision was made to use the words "ought" and "must," the latter to express exceptionless norms and the former a normative recommendation to which individual ethics committees might seek to justify permitting exceptions.

By accepting that there are occasions when an exceptionless norm is appropriate, signified by the use of "must," AHEC gave effect to the idea that good may not be achieved by acts that destroy that which is good or which cause harm to individual members of the human family. In effect AHEC thus adopted a secular version of the Pauline principle, or at least a pluralist principle that seemed to express the same idea.

I see this process of expressing morality in a pluralist environment as a good activity, one that seeks to identify and protect human beings.

It does this from a viewpoint that listens to the different faiths, cultures and traditions within our society and seeks to reflect the committee's perceptions of what needs to be protected in the conduct of human research and health care clinical practices, in the light of values that are derived from the society but transcend its cultural and traditional differences. One of my most valuable experiences in that respect was the development through consultation of guidelines for conducting research with Aboriginal and Torres Strait Islander people. The set of core values that were described seemed to contain a depth of meaning and express a greater sense of community than had otherwise been developed in NHMRC documents.

Most importantly, as I have described it, the NHMRC process does not exclude views, but in fact is required by statute law to be inclusive in its membership and responsive to public consultation in its processes. It is therefore something of a model for the formation of public policy in tolerant, inclusive, pluralist Australian society.

The Australian society of which I am proud to be a part is not a society that rejects the contribution of the religious or the non-religious; it welcomes all contributions and is confident enough in its processes to be open to suggestions from every tradition and culture, and prepared to evaluate each suggestion for its worth and merit in the shared task of pursuing the common good, doing so in a way that is respectful of the worth and dignity of every member of the human family.

Crucial to the notion of a democracy is not only government *by* the people, but also *for* the people. That a decision reflects the majority view does not in itself make the decision democratic. Majorities can make undemocratic decisions. A majority decision that fails to respect a minority, or fails to respect and protect each individual member of the human family, would not be a decision *for* the people and hence would be undemocratic.

6

Teaching and Learning Constructive Critical Evaluation[210]

6.1 Applying the Australian Qualifications Framework in Bioethics

The graduate courses in Bioethics that I teach are designed for those who are professionally engaged in the medical, nursing or biological sciences, law, social sciences or education, who wish to further their understanding of moral decision-making and ethical policy in those disciplines, or take leadership in ensuring that the new technologies serve humanity. Some of those who take the courses are already members of ethics committees and take a graduate course to equip them better for that task. Graduates may be prepared to become members of ethics committees or they may occupy leadership positions within their own institutions or discipline. Some may teach. Some may go on to become academics.

The Australian Qualifications Framework[211] requires that Masters graduates are able to:

- provide appropriate evidence of advanced knowledge

---

[210] This paper is reproduced with permission from where it was first published in *Ethics Education* Volume 16, No. 2, 2010.
[211] Australian Qualification Framework accessed 21/8/08 at http://www.aqf.edu.au/pdf/han51_72.pdf.

about a specialist body of theoretical and applied topics;
- demonstrate a high order of skill in analysis, critical evaluation and/or professional application through the planning and execution of project work or a piece of scholarship or research; and
- demonstrate creativity and flexibility in the application of knowledge and skills to new situations, to solve complex problems and to think rigorously and independently.

The skills of *analysis* and *critical evaluation* differ from one discipline to another. How they are done in mathematics differs from how they are done in history, for example. The question that I have been seeking to answer for my own students is basically, how can they learn those skills and, more to the point, how can I assist them to learn those skills in the area of Bioethics? Learning the ability to demonstrate creativity and flexibility in the application of knowledge and skills to new situations raises similar questions.

Thinking about the skill set has made me reflect critically on my own teaching and on the assessment tasks that the students complete and whether in fact the assessment assesses their ability to apply that skill set constructively in the environments in which they are likely to be engaged. This reflection uncovered a gap between what I was teaching and the skills that I apply in my involvement in ethics committees and at the level of assisting to form Government policy[212].

6.2   Gatekeepers in Biomedicine

Sixteen years ago, Renee Fox and Judith Swazey, two counsellors who had worked in the field of organ replacement for many years, including with the Jarvik 7 artificial heart experiments and through the period of the development of successful organ transplantation, described the

---

[212] The author was a member of the Australian health Ethics Committee, a Principal Committee of the NHMRC and of several other NHMRC committees (chairing two) and of the Ethics Panel of the Victorian Infertility Treatment Authority.

role of ethical "gatekeepers" in Biomedicine.[213] They described three levels of gatekeeping.

The *primary gatekeepers* included those involved in initiating and carrying out a procedure: clinicians and medical researchers, and patients and their families.

The *secondary gatekeepers* included those not directly making the decision but able to influence the decision or whose authority or permission may be required such as:

- senior hospital and university administrators;
- human research ethics committees;
- clinical practice committees;
- medical colleges and professional peers;
- legislators, courts, government and statutory review authorities (e.g. in Australia the National Health and Medical Research Council, Office of the Gene Technology Regulator, Therapeutic Goods Administration, State Reproductive Technology Councils).

Tertiary gatekeepers included those not *directly* involved in making or influencing decisions but who shape opinions, such as: professional journals; expert analysts and commentators in health law, medical ethics, social science and health policy; and the print and electronic media.

As the technology continued to develop, the discipline of Bioethics developed as a response to the need for there to be people who are professionally trained in understanding the complex ethical issues that have been spawned by the technology. Training in Bioethics became an area of interest for those in the health professions and is now a normal part of training in a health profession, with some health professionals and health administrators choosing to take study in the area further.

---

[213] Renee C Fox and Judith P Swazey, *Spare Parts: Organ Replacement in American Society* (Oxford: OUP, 1992), pp 178-189.

6.3 Constructivism is a Natural Outcome

One of the most enjoyable aspects of teaching at graduate level is the students' level of professional resources and life experience. In a class of doctors, other health professionals and others from a wider range of professional experience, there is no shortage of case examples for Bioethics problems from the students' own experience. The challenge for a teacher is to evoke those experiences, because this makes the learning experience far more successful not only for the student whose experiences are being discussed, but also for others taking part in the discussion. It is a process in which they are actively engaged.[214] Such discussion is also likely to be focussed on problem solving rather than highlighting difference.

In teaching analysis, part of the process is undoubtedly teaching students to identify difference and in Bioethics that boils down to teaching them about metaethics and philosophical anthropology, the impact of the latter on the nature of moral theory, and then the different types of normative theory, then applying those theories in practice to show the different outcomes. Thus the analysis of a case discussion at the applied level can go back to differences at each of the other levels.[215]

Part of the process of being constructive is not to set out to dismiss any view, but to seek out and recognise goodness wherever it is, rather than to seek out difference and to dismiss error. In a classroom situation

---

[214] John Biggs and Catherine Tang, *Teaching for Quality Learning at University* 3rd Edition 2007, p.10.

[215] "*Metaethics* investigates where our ethical principles come from, and what they mean. Are they merely social inventions? Do they involve more than expressions of our individual emotions? Metaethical answers to these questions focus on the issues of universal truths, the will of God, the role of reason in ethical judgments, and the meaning of ethical terms themselves. *Normative ethics* takes on a more practical task, which is to arrive at moral standards that regulate right and wrong conduct. This may involve articulating the good habits that we should acquire, the duties that we should follow, or the consequences of our behavior on others. Finally, *applied ethics* involves examining specific controversial issues, such as abortion, infanticide, animal rights, environmental concerns, homosexuality, capital punishment, or nuclear war." (*Encyclopedia of Philosophy* 2008).

when confronted by a particular case, students will mostly attempt to find points of agreement rather than wanting to pursue disagreement. In written work however the outcome tends to be very different. They tend to *slash and burn* alternative views. To be fair, the assessment process that I experienced as a student and which I had been applying to my students did not evaluate the ability to use understanding of difference constructively, only destructively in a kind of winner-take-all approach to analysis. The teaching of essay writing tended to produce combativeness rather than constructiveness. In other words, it seems that constructivism is the natural approach for-face to-face discussion and divisive analysis is learned to fulfil the requirements for written assessment. The challenge is to assist students to undertake analysis constructively.

6.4 Experimenting with Active Learning

In trying to engage students in active participation in the classroom, one of the approaches I had adopted was a classroom debate which was done for assessment. To reduce the disadvantage of students who were not good at oral presentation, they were asked to submit their own presentation notes for the debate at the start of the session and their assessment took the written component into account. The teams were allocated randomly by simply taking every second person seated in the classroom one day to be a team (well, almost randomly - one year there were two husband and wife teams that it seemed important to separate), and the affirmative and negative teams chosen by coin toss. The debates were held on major public issues and were a public performance with faculty members attending in academic dress, the formality of a professional adjudicator and chaired by the Director of the institute. A disproportionate amount of work usually went into the debates, as far as I could see, with much team work on display, and they were colourful occasions. The individual assessments were not made known publicly, just the team results.

Thus for instance, a debate held in a class on a course called "End of

Life Ethics" was on the topic "That euthanasia should be legalised."

For that debate the affirmative side was given a number of sub-propositions and asked to choose which they would use, allocating a speaker to each chosen topic, and notifying the negative team immediately of which propositions were to be used. The sub-propositions were:

1. If society recognises the autonomy of individuals by granting them the right to pursue their views about the good life and create their own lives, then the logical consequence is to allow people to decide their own death.
2. Since one of the main aims of medicine is to relieve suffering, it is a medical duty to relieve the intractable suffering of a patient by assisting her to die.
3. The sacredness of human life is a religious belief. The law should not enforce religious beliefs. When there is a division in society between the right to die with dignity and religious claims about the sanctity of human life, legislation that prohibits assistance to die for a person who is so ill that she can no longer enjoy life and wants to die is undemocratic and unjust.
4. There is a difference between the physical or biological life and the biographical life – that which gives it meaning, for example dreams, aspirations, achievements etc. If that is lost, then there is no person because they have lost their distinctive value. The sanctity of life no longer applies to a human that has lost all the characteristics that make it a person.
5. Human life is sacred. The value of human life should not be degraded by reducing the quality of life for the sake of extending the quantity of life. When a person has no quality of life, then she should be able to choose to die.
6. Withdrawal of life-saving treatment is permissible under

the law. The effect of such a decision is the same as administering a fatal treatment. The two acts are morally indistinguishable. In fact, administering a fatal treatment would often be more humane than starving someone to death, letting them die of dehydration or letting them drown in their sputum through not treating pneumonia. The law should be consistent.

7. The arguments against euthanasia are mainly slippery-slope arguments. Euthanasia legislation can be drafted so that the practice is safe.

I have described this assessment item in detail because even though it was popular and successful in terms of displaying and evaluating student skills, I have more recently questioned whether it is actually testing skills that are advantageous, given the likely circumstances in which the students will find themselves. It is developing and testing their ability to hold and defend a position in peer discussion, and that is one of the expected learning objectives. Also the process of working together in a team and the coaching that goes on between team members is an intensely active learning experience. However, it is a process that is based on magnifying difference rather than on constructive evaluation. In that respect, perhaps it teaches at least some to have a better understanding of a view other than there own and that may be constructive. But overall it does not take them to the next step, which is to use their ability to understand differences between moral positions constructively in order to work towards a consensus. The debate showed the skills of demolition, not necessarily the skills of building a rapport between people of different views. The skills that they showed are not necessarily the skills that I would want on display at a committee that I was chairing or in a head of department or in a clinician dealing with complex decisions with a patient or patient's family.

6.5 Developing a Learning Outcome for Constructive Critical Evaluation

That observation raises a question about how one ought to evaluate the Bioethics needs of the health sector and thus determine the desired qualities and skills that may be required of Bioethics graduates who will serve that sector. Based on my own experience, someone who can take critical analysis from exploring and evaluating difference towards constructive solutions to the issues raised will better serve the health sector than someone who stops at the level of simply arguing over differences. There is a need for something more than polemics.

Expressing this as a desirable learning outcome would read something like:

- Demonstrate the ability to undertake analysis and critical evaluation constructively and creatively to achieve maximum contribution of others in the development of broadly acceptable solutions.

In approaching critical analysis with students, this goal has led me to seek to have them identify not the weaknesses in a moral position that they are studying, but its strengths – to put it simply, to identify goodness and virtue rather than error and vice.

The desirable learning outcome would in itself seem to be motivating, first, because the outcome is obviously desirable in relation to the needs of the workplace, and second, because such a skill would be valued by others. It would be motivating also because it would be a personal achievement, and finally because trying to achieve it ought to be fun. Thus it would seem to fulfil the four levels of motivation that Biggs and Tang describe: extrinsic, social, achievement and intrinsic.[216]

Excellent teaching of ethics along these lines would assist the graduate to be a useful contributor to policy formation in a way that respects the differences of participants and assists each to express

---

[216] John Biggs and Catherine Tang, *Teaching for Quality Learning at University* 3rd Edition 2007 p. 34.

ideal solutions to problems from their own culture and professional experience.

6.6 Challenges to Constructive Critical Evaluation

That there can be inclusive solutions in Bioethics is open to challenge. In discussion about Bioethics and issues in Bioethics, there are some common moral discussion stoppers; claims such as:

a) People disagree on solutions to moral issues.
b) Who am I to judge others?
c) Morality is a private matter.
d) Morality is simply a matter for individual cultures to decide.

Claims such as these foster the view that no policy on moral questions is achievable because no consensus is achievable.

People usually initially disagree on solutions to moral issues, but the point of moral discussion is to explore the differences, rather than to see difference as either necessary or unresolvable. There is something very adolescent about seeing difference of view as the end rather than the beginning of discussion. Experts in many areas disagree on key issues in their fields, but that is why they publish scientific findings and hold scientific conferences. The differences do not stop the progress of science and nor should they stop the progress of moral discussion.

Despite differences of perspectives, and different belief structures and starting points, we are all dealing with the same human reality. The international human rights movement attests to the fact that there are many moral issues on which people agree, and there are values that transcend or are common across cultures and religions. I found participation in the development of UNESCO's *Universal Declaration on the Human Genome and Human Rights*[217] an engaging experience

---

[217] *Universal Declaration on the Human Genome and Human Rights* 1997 http://portal.unesco.org/shs/en/ev.php-URL_ID=1881&URL_DO=DO_TOPIC&URL_SECTION=201.html.

precisely because it showed that on such a difficult topic, diverse peoples and cultures could transcend their differences.

It is also the case that disagreements may not be about substantial moral beliefs, but about non-moral facts of a matter, or simply about participation in the common project that we call a community.

The question, "Who am I to judge others?" is important but misdirected. Tolerance of others and their moral decisions is important. In health care a patient may refuse a treatment and not wish to discuss the matter further. That privacy is their right. However, most often patients seek to discuss their decisions, looking for assistance with obtaining the necessary information, and seeking the health professional's opinion not just on the medical facts but also on what are often complex moral choices. Sometimes there is disagreement over values, and sometimes the disagreement is such that as a matter of conscience, the health professional respectfully withdraws from care because what is being asked conflicts with his or her own convictions. But the health professional or the patient deciding whether something is the right course of action is not the same thing as judging a person. There is also a distinction between judging as condemning and judging as evaluating, and disagreement over the right course of action is distinct from a judgement about either of the persons involved.

The claim that morality is a private matter is often intended to stop discussion. Privacy is an important right, and people are entitled to keep their counsel about their relationships and intimacies. There is no obligation to participate in moral discussion, and privacy in health care is particularly important. However a common morality is what establishes and to an extent defines an institution or a professional group as a community and enables it to share common purpose in both policy and action. Some aspects of morality are thus essentially public. Even a social or sporting club needs commonly accepted rules of conduct. In relating to one another, we need conventions about behaviour and social expectations. Further, being able to discuss and to reason about morality is important and allows us to recognize the harm that some of our choices may cause. Moral choices are often not isolated personal preferences, but are to do with interpersonal relationships and living in community.

The relativist claim that morality is simply a matter for individual cultures to decide is a confusion between describing a morality and adopting a morality. There are moral principles that transcend culture because they are based on shared human reality. We need to be able to discern whether a cultural practice should be changed, such as the cultural practice of female genital mutilation. Policy reform would be impossible if we were to take the view that culture is beyond criticism.

The education of the so-called Y-generation by baby boomers seems to have given them a strong sense of positivism, that is, the belief that meaningful statements are either empirically verifiable (e.g., HIV causes AIDS) or analytic truths (e.g., one cannot make a round square). The new generation (generation Y) appears to be positivist in that it tends to assert that value judgements are neither empirically verifiable nor analytic truths. They are merely expressions of feeling or emotions. In that, they tend to make a distinction between prescriptive and descriptive meaning. Values, they would claim, must not be confused with facts.

The conviction that there are no moral truths does not exclude the development of some moral convictions. If you begin with the belief that all moral beliefs are entirely subjective, just feelings, then you will crave some kind of rule for resolving all those differences of opinion. One such rule is a basic notion of consistency. This generation believes strongly in the injustice of discrimination. They want moral and policy decisions to apply equally to like situations. This is the principle of universalisability: if I hold that something is wrong in one situation, I must hold that it is also wrong in all relevantly similar situations.

This leads to what might be called universalised prescriptivism: the right moral judgement or policy is that which treats everyone's preferences as equally important and then seeks simply to do the best to satisfy as many preferences as possible, giving weight to the relative strength of preferences. This is preference utilitarianism[218] and varies only slightly from classical utilitarianism, which taught that one should maximize happiness by maximizing pleasure and minimizing pain. A major problem with applying a principle of universalizability in this way is that it ignores what is often called the separateness of persons[219] or the difference principle.[220] Utilitarianism aggregates happiness or preferences without regard to the relative inequalities that may occur in maximizing total or average preference satisfaction or total or average happiness. Universilisabilty could also be used to justify doing the best by the worst off, which is an outcome of what Rawls refers to as the separateness persons.[221]

In responding constructively to a person who seeks to direct a committee along utilitarian lines, one can make the usual attacks on the position, such as that utilitarianism is an aggregative theory and fails to acknowledge the "separateness of persons."[222] It focuses on overall consequences and not on the individual. A person's moral identity is constituted by his or her commitments and moral integrity in relationship with others, for which utilitarianism has no explanation. In utilitarianism my identity is subsumed into a kind of single personhood. There is also no accounting for how my preferences are formed. The preferences of Mother Theresa and Saddam Hussein rank the same in the calculation. This approach, by focussing on consequences, ignores the virtues of agents and the fact that choices to act shape the identity of who I am. If I steal, I make myself a thief; if I kill, I make myself a murderer; in giving to another, I make myself a lover.

A more constructive approach to the utilitarian committee member

---

[218] For a formal account of this basis for preference utilitarianism see R.M. Hare, *Moral Thinking: Its Levels, Method and Point Method* (Oxford: Oxford University Press 1981).

[219] John Rawls in *A Theory of Justice*, rev. ed. (Cambridge, MA: Belknap Press of Harvard University Press 1999).

220 John Rawls, "The Independence of Moral Theory" *Proceedings and Addresses of the American Philosophical Association* Volume 47, No. 5 p. 22, in *Collected Papers* 1999 pp. 286-302.

[221] Ibid.

[222] Ibid.

might be to avoid the metaethical claims about universalizability and talk about the value of non-discrimination and avoiding arbitrariness. After all, if one had to choose between an allegedly "logical" requirement of any ethical view, and the avoidance of discrimination and arbitrary treatment of others, the latter may have stronger claims on us. From that agreed basis one could hope then to move the other to seeing the importance of first addressing the needs of the worst off rather than aggregating benefits.[223]

In this discussion, I have tried to show the difference between critical evaluation that is dismissive, and critical evaluation that constructively uses knowledge of the positive attributes and the deficiencies, acknowledging that the positive provides a platform for moving to a better developed position.

Similarly, for a committee member who makes categorical statements about the rightness or wrongness of a particular ethical choice (what is sometimes called deontology or even fundamentalist), the solution is to seek out what it is that he or she wants to protect by making the claim, and to encourage that to be asserted as something good or valued. That then makes sense to others without losing altogether what the person expressed, and it provides some substance for debate other than dismissal by either side.

We need some basic notions to make better sense of ethics. First, ethics is prescriptive – that is what defines it. It is about deciding what is right and what is wrong in a given situation. Second, moral norms are universalisable – that is a logical requirement of making the same judgement in relevantly similar circumstances. The present generation is right in recognising that ethics should be consistent and not discriminatory or arbitrary. Third, ethics is about freely chosen actions. We are responsible for our own choices (taking into account positive responsibilities to act and to be informed and acknowledging the complications of involuntariness). Fourth, ethics is agent-centred—

---

[223] This paragraph was suggested by a reviewer J O Quilter 12/12/09 and I am grateful for that and several other comments offered by him and by the second reviewer that improved the paper, especially its readability.

about the agent as well as about the outcome of the agent's actions. When we choose to act we create the person we are. When we act wrongly, we do so by acting contrary to the goodness of the human person. In that sense, a wrong act is essentially a contradictory act in that it is an act against or neglecting what is good. Fifth, ethics is descriptive – it describes the agent's commitments (whether sentimental, rational, autonomous, heteronomous (determined by others), or in a theological context heteronomously theonomous (determined by God), or participatively theonomous[224] (determined by our participation in God's love). Otherwise from a philosophical perspective ethics has no content.

The paradox for ethical theory lies in being both descriptive and universalisable. The desire to resolve the paradox is what drives moral conversation. In ethical discussion we tend to seek a solution that is universalisable, prescriptive, descriptive, agent-centred, and free.

6.7 Problem-based Learning and Constructive Critical Evaluation

In my own teaching experience, constructivism is the natural outcome in a problem-solving environment, and what is needed to achieve the learning outcome of *constructive critical evaluation* is to learn to undertake critical evaluation within a constructive context. My good students learned to be critical and to evaluate, but they needed to learn to take those skills a step further, to use them as a basis for working with others towards a broadly acceptable outcome.

One of my richest experiences is to have sat on a national committee that was required to undertake public consultation at each stage of the process of developing ethical guidelines. The NHMRC is required by its statute to undertake public consultation in the development of

---

[224] *Veritatis Splendor.*

ethical guidelines.²²⁵ The usual process is to develop and publish an Issues Paper that identifies the scope of the issue to be considered, and to send that out for what is called a targeted consultation, usually targeted to those who have a professional interest in the area. The submissions are used to develop a draft set of guidelines, which are then sent out for public consultation. A second draft is then prepared and sent out for a final round of public consultation.

The process of developing guidelines is thus cautious, but more importantly, the double process of public consultation encourages the committee to respond to the expectations expressed in the submissions and so develop a document that is broadly acceptable. The experience is enormously educative and thus privileged. From many disparate views, the committee is expected to develop a single outcome and it is answerable for how it achieves that.

As a teacher of Bioethics, my task is to create a learning experience that in some way matches that experience. The submissions to public bodies such as the NHMRC are usually available, and they provide a ready source of material. One learning approach is to select some of the many submissions and set a group of student the task of working from the submissions to an outcome on a particular issue.

For instance, one of the major issues in reproductive technology is pre-implantation genetic diagnosis (PGD). In 2004, the NHMRC promulgated *Ethical guidelines on the use of assisted reproductive technology in clinical practice and research*.²²⁶ The guidelines were reissued in 2007 with changes to accommodate the cloning legislation. Compliance by Australian IVF teams with the guidelines is secured by the terms of the funding agreements with the Commonwealth and by the administration of standards by the Reproductive Technology Accreditation Committee.

The guidelines require that PGD of embryos must not be used for:

---

²²⁵ National Health and Medical Research Council Act 1992 section 12 accessed 22/5/08 at http://www.comlaw.gov.au/ComLaw/Legislation/ActCompilation1.nsf/0/23029FDD3FCC3FD7CA25719C008331D3/$file/NatHeaMedResCou1992WD02.pdf.
²²⁶ Available from http://www.nhmrc.gov.au/publications/synopses/e78syn.htm.

- prevention of conditions that do not seriously harm the person to be born;
- selection of the sex of an embryo except to reduce the risk of transmission of a serious genetic condition; or
- selection in favour of a genetic defect or disability in the person to be born.

This restriction may challenge those who uphold the notions of *reproductive rights* and *reproductive freedom*, especially those who are of the view that it is their right to choose the sex or other genetic features of their child. There are also those who favour using PGD to choose a "saviour sibling" so that that child's tissue may be used to treat an older existing child. The NHMRC received submissions from people who held those views, and from others who took a "rights of the child" view.

What counts as serious harm is also open to debate. There are those who argue that in a family who already have a child who is autistic, IVF and PGD for sex selection is permissible in order to have a girl rather than a boy because studies have shown that a boy would be four times more likely to be autistic.

IVF practitioners also raise questions about whether they can withhold IVF from a person who is, for instance, a convicted paedophile or from someone who already has other children who have been taken into care.

The overall rationale adopted by the NHMRC for restricting choice in the use of reproductive technology is that "Clinical decisions must respect, primarily, the interests and welfare of the persons who may be born, as well as the long-term health and psychosocial welfare of all participants, including gamete donors"[227]

The jurisprudential dialogue about reproductive rights occurs against a background of the legal tradition that the interests of the child are paramount. This principle found expression in the UN *Convention*

---

[227] NHMRC *Ethical guidelines on the use of assisted reproductive technology in clinical practice and research* 2007 p. 9, available from http://www.nhmrc.gov.au/publications/synopses/e78syn.htm.

on the Rights of the Child,[228] which recognizes, amongst other matters, the rights of the child to an identity, nationality, family relations, and to personal relations and direct contact with both parents. In this respect too, family law has been based on the notion that the interests of the child are paramount. Family law restricts parental choices and resolves conflicts in favour of the welfare of children.

The group of students may therefore be provided with a set of submissions representing the range of views on such an issue and asked to develop ethical guidelines. Each individual is then asked to write a rationale for each of the guidelines adopted by the group and how the submissions were taken into account, and they are assessed on the rationale. They develop the guidelines in their own time and during that period, they are attending lectures. The group task makes the students much more active in discussion, as they see the critical analysis of different approaches to ethics provided in the lectures as a resource for their assessment task.

The approach uses both group work and problem-based learning and the assessment task is both a learning device and an adequate assessment tool. The task engages them in critical evaluation and in using that critical evaluation constructively.

The object of this approach is for the members of an ethics committee to see their task as seeking to guide relationships between clinicians and patients, researchers and research participants as an ideal. Ideally the relationship protects the development and flourishing of the patient/participant and the ethics committee's function is to assist by identifying the elements of human flourishing that may be at risk. By pursuing what is best in relationships it is proves much easier to reach consensus than the common alternative for ethics committees which is to seek a level of consensus on what might not be tolerated.

---

[228] Available from: http://www2.ohchr.org/english/law/crc.htm.

Bibliography

Aquinas, Thomas, *In Duo Praecepta Caritatis et in Decem Legis Praecepta. De Dilectione Dei: Opuscula Theologica*, II, No. 1168, Ed. Taurinen, 1954.

Aquinas, Thomas, *Quaestiones Quodlibetales*, Spiazzi, Raimondo M. (ed.) Torino: Marietti, 1956.

Aquinas, Thomas, *Summa Theologiae*, Thomas Gilby (General editor), Garden City: Image Books, 1969.

Augustine, "The Enchiridion" in Philip Schaff (ed). *Augustine: On the Holy Trinity, Doctrinal treatises, Moral treatises*, Peabody: Hendrickson, 1994.

Australian Bureau of Statistics, *Marriages Australia 2005*, Document No. 3306.0.55.001.

Beauchamp, Tom, L, James F. Childress, *Principles of Biomedical Ethics* (5th Edition) New York: OUP, 2001.

Benedict XVI, Pope, *Deus Caritas Est*, 2005.

Biggs, John and Catherine Tang, *Teaching for Quality Learning at University*, 3rd Edition, London: McGraw-Hill, 2007.

Black v. The Commonwealth (1981) HCA 2, (1981) 146 CLR 559 (2 February 1981), at 579,

Bowie, Norman and Tom Beauchamp, *Ethical Theory in Business*, Englewood Cliffs: Prentice-Hall, 1979.

Center for Holocaust and Genocide Studies, University of Minnesota.

Churchill, Sir Winston, Letter from to Lord Asquith, December 1910, http://www.winstonchurchill.org/support/the-churchill-centre/publications/finest-hour-online/594-churchill-and-eugenics.

Congregation for the Doctrine of the Faith, *Dignitas Personae*, 2008.

Congregation for the Doctrine of the Faith, *Instruction Donum Vitae*, 1988.

Control Council Law No. 10, Punishment of Persons Guilty of War Crimes, Crimes Against Peace and Against Humanity, December 20, 1945, 3 *Official Gazette Control Council for Germany* 50-55 (1946). http://www1.umn.edu/humanrts/instree/ccno10.htm

Comfort, Nathaniel, "The prisoner as model organism: malaria research at Stateville.

Convention on the Rights of People with Disabilities http://www.un.org/disabilities/convention/conventionfull.shtml.

Dworkin, Ronald, *Life's Dominion*, New York: Knopf, 1993.

Emanuel, Linda L. ed. *Regulating How We Die: The Ethical, Medical, and Legal Issues Surrounding Physician-Assisted Suicide*, Cambridge: Harvard University Press. 1998.

Engber-Perdersen, Troels, *Paul and the Stoics*, Edinburgh: T&T Clark, 2000.

European Commission, "Social values, Science and Technology" Eurobarometer 2005, http://ec.europa.eu/public_opinion/archives/ebs/ebs_225_report_en.pdf.

Eyster, Zachary C., *Imagining ethics: re-imagining salvation: Josef Fuchs, fundamental option, and the soteriological implications thereof,* Villanova University, 2009.

Finnis, John, *Moral Absolutes: Tradition, Revision, and Truth,* Washington DC: Catholic University of America Press, 1991.

Finnis, John M., Germain G. Grisez, & Joseph M. Boyle, "'Direct' and 'Indirect': A Reply to Critics of Our Action Theory". *Thomist.* Vol. 65, No. 1, 2001, pp. 1-44.

Finnis, John N., *Fundamentals of Ethics,* Oxford: University Press, 1983.

Fitzmeyer SJ, Joseph A., *Paul and his Theology: A Brief Sketch*, New Jersey: Prentice Hall, 1989.

Fleming, John and Nicholas Tonti-Filippini (eds.), *Common Ground? Seeking an Asutralian Consensus on Abortion and Sex Education*, Strathfield: St Paul Publications, 2007.

Fletcher, Joseph, "Ethics and Euthanasia" in Emanuel, Linda L. (ed.) *Regulating How We Die: The Ethical, Medical, and Legal Issues Surrounding Physician-Assisted Suicide*, Cambridge: Harvard University Press, 1998.

Fletcher, Joseph, *The Ethics of Genetic Control: Ending Reproductive Roulette*, New York: Doubleday and Company, 1974.

Fletcher, Joseph, *Hello Lovers: An Introduction to Situation Ethics*, (with Thomas A. Wassmer SJ). New York: Corpus Books & World, 1970.

Fletcher, Joseph, *Moral Responsibility: Situation Ethics at Work*, Philadelphia: Westminster Press, 1967.

Fletcher, Joseph, *Morals and Medicine*, New Jersey: Princeton University Press, 1954.

Fletcher, Joseph, *Situation Ethics: The New Morality*, Philadelphia: Westminster Press, 1966.

Fletcher, Joseph, *The Situation Ethics Debate* (with Harvey Cox), Philadelphia: Westminster Press, 1968.

Fletcher, Joseph, *Situation Ethics: True or False* (with John Montgomery), Minneapolis: Dimension Books, 1972.

Foot, Philippa, *The Problem of Abortion and the Doctrine of the Double Effect* in *Virtues and Vices*, Oxford: Basil Blackwell, 1978.

Fox, Renee C. and Judith P Swazey, *Spare Parts: Organ Replacement in American Society*, Oxford: OUP, 1992,

Fuchs, Joseph, "The Absoluteness of Behavioural Moral Norms", *Gregorianum*, 1971 cf. Zachary C. Eyster, *Imagining ethics: re-imagining salvation: Josef Fuchs, fundamental option, and the soteriological implications thereof* Villanova University, 2009.

Grisez, Germain et al, *Abortion: The Myths, the Realities and the Arguments,* Washington: Corpus Books, 1970.

Grisez, Germain, "Faith, Philosophy and Fidelity", *Fidelity,* Volume 3, No. 8, July 1984.

Grisez, Germain, "The True and Ultimate End of Human Beings: The kingdom, Not God Alone", *Theological Studies,* Vol. 69, 2008: pp. 38-61.

Grisez, Germain, *The Way of the Lord Jesus Volume 2, Christian Moral Principles,* Chicago: Franciscan Herald Press, 1983.

Hare, Richard M., *Moral Thinking, its Level, Method and Point,* Oxford: OUP, 1981.

Herman, Barbara, *The Practice of Moral Judgement,* Cambridge: Harvard University Press, 1993.

Hill, Thomas E. Jnr., *Dignity and Practical Reason in Kant's Moral Theory,* Ithaca: Cornell University Press, 1992.

Hitler, Adolf, *Letter to Reishsleiter Bouhler and Dr. med. Brandt,* September 1, 1939, http://constitutionalistnc.tripod.com/hitler-leftist/id16.html.

Hogan, Michael, "Separation of Church and State?", May 16, 2001, http://www.australianreview.net/digest/2001/05/hogan.html.

Hoyt, Robert (ed.) *The Birth-Control Debate,* Kansas City: The National Catholic Reporter, 1969.

International Covenant on Civil and Political Rights, http://www2.ohchr.org/english/law.

International Covenants on Economic, Social and Cultural Rights. http://www2.ohchr.org/english/law.

International Theological Commission, *The Search for a Universal Ethic* 2009, translation by Joseph Bolin, March 9, 2010, www.pathsoflove.com/universal-ethics-natural-law.html. The official French and Italian versions are available at http://www.vatican.va/roman_curia/congregations/cfaith/cti_index.htm.

John Paul II, Pope, *Evangelium Vitae*, 1995

John Paul II, Pope, *Fides et Ratio*, 1998.

John Paul II, Pope, *The Theology of the Body: Human Love in the Divine Plan*, Boston: Pauline Books & Media, 1997.

John Paul II, Pope *Veritatis Splendor*, 1993.

Journet, Charles, *The Meaning of Grace*, London: Chapman, 1960.

Kant, Immanuel, *The Grounding of the Metaphysics of Morality*, tr. James W Ellington, Indianapolis: Hackett Publishing Company, 1981.

Kerr, Fergus, *Twentieth Century Catholic Theologian*, Blackwell: Oxford, 2007.

Knauer, Peter, "The Hermeneutic Function of the Double Effect Reasoning," first published in French in 1965 and in English in the journal *Natural Law Forum*, Vol. 12, 1967: pp. 132-62.

Leo XIII, Pope, *Libertas Praestantissimum*, 1888.

McCormick, Richard, "Ambiguity in Moral Choice" in McCormick, Richard and Paul Ramsey, *Doing Evil to Achieve Good: Moral Choice in Conflict Situations*, Chicago: Loyola University, 1978.

McCormick, Richard, "Classification Through Dialogue" in McCormick, Richard and Charles Curran, *The Historical Development of Moral Theology in the United States*, New Jersey: Paulist Press, 1999.

McCormick, Richard and Paul Ramsey, *Doing Evil to Achieve Good: Moral Choice in Conflict Situations*, Chicago: Loyola University, 1978.

McCormick, Richard, *How Brave a New World? Dilemmas in Bioethics*, New York: Doubleday, 1985.

McCormick, Richard and Charles Curran, *The Historical Development of Moral Theology in the United States*, New Jersey: Paulist Press, 1999.

McCormick, Richard, "The Question is not Closed," in Hoyt, Robert (ed.) *The Birth-Control Debate*, Kansas City: The National Catholic Reporter, 1969.

MacIntyre, Alasdair, *After Virtue*, Notre Dame: University of Notre Dame Press, 1981.

Macintyre, Alasdair "Moral Relativism, Truth and Justification" in his *The Task of Philosophy Vol. 1*. Cambridge: Cambridge University Press 2006.

MacIntyre, Alasdair *The Task of Philosophy Vol. 1*, Cambridge: Cambridge University Press, 2006.

MacIntyre, Alasdair *Whose Justice, Which Rationality*, London: Duckworth, 1988.

May, William E. *Moral Theologians and Veritatis Splendor,* http://www.ewtn.com/library/THEOLOGY/MORALVS.HTM.

Mill, John Stuart, *Essay on Liberty*, [S.l.]: Megalodon Entertainment, 2008.

Mitchell, Alex, "Faulkner Lone State ALP Senator to Back Cloning Legislation," *The Sun Herald*, November 12 2006, p. 22.

National Institutes of Health, *Regulations and Ethical Guidelines*. http://ohsr.od.nih.gov/guidelines/belmont.html#ethical.

National Health and Medical Research Council, *Organ and Tissue Donation by Living Donors: Guidelines for Ethical Practice for health Professionals* Endorsed 15 March 2007; *Organ and Tissue Donation after Death, for Transplantation: Guidelines for Ethical Practice by Health Professionals.* Endorsed 15 March 2007.

National Health and Medical Research Council, *Ethical Guidelines for the Care of People in Post Coma Unresponsiveness (Vegetative State) or a Minimally Responsive State*, Australian Government Canberra 2008, http://www.nhmrc.gov.au/publications/synopses/e81_82syn.htm.

National Health and Medical Research Council, *National Statement on Ethical Conduct in Human Research* Australian Government Canberra 2007.

National Health and Medical Research Council, *Ethical guidelines on the use of assisted reproductive technology in clinical practice and research* 2007 http://www.nhmrc.gov.au/publications/synopses/e78syn.htm.

Nikzor Project, The, http://www.nizkor.org/ftp.cgi/places/ftp.py?places//germany/euthanasia/brandt.001.

Novak, M. "Human dignity, human rights", *First Things*, 97 (November) 1999: pp.39-42.

O'Malley, John W., *Four Cultures of the West*, London: Harvard University Press, 2004.

Papal Commission on Birth Control *The Tablet* 22nd April 1967 pp. 449-454; April 29th 1967 pp. 478-485; 6th May 1967 pp. 510-513; 21 September 1968 pp. 949-951.

Pell, George Cardinal, "Varieties of Intolerance: Religious and Secular", Inaugural Hilary Term Lecture, Oxford University Newman Society, The Divinity School, Oxford University, March 9, 2009.

Pius XII, Pope, "Allocution on 'New Morality'," April 19, 1952, *Acta Apostolica Sedis*, Vol. 44, 1952.

Porter, Jean, "'Direct' and 'Indirect' in Grisez's Moral Theory", *Theological Studies*, Vol. 57, 1996: p. 612.

Rahner S.J., Karl *Foundations of Christian Faith: An Introduction to the Idea of Christianity*, trans. William V. Dych, New York: Seabury Press, 1978: p. 93–106.

Rahner SJ, Karl, "Theology of Freedom," *Theological Investigations, Vol. 6, Concerning Vatican Council II*, trans. Karl-H. and Boniface Kruger, Baltimore: Helicon, 1969: pp. 178–93.

Rahner SJ, Karl, *Theological Investigations, Volume 5, Later Writings*, trans. Karl-H. Kruger, Baltimore: Helicon 1966: pp. 445–51.

Ratzinger, Cardinal Joseph An address to the Congregation of the Doctrine of the Faith, "Current Situation of Faith and Theology" 1996, http://www.ourladyswarriors.org/dissent/ratzsitu596.htm.

Ratzinger, Joseph Cardinal, *Conscience and Truth*, Presented at the 10th Workshop for Bishops, February 1991, Dallas, Texas, http://www.ewtn.com/library/curia/ratzcons.htm.

Ratzinger, Joseph Cardinal, in "Faith, Religion and Culture" in *Truth and Tolerance*, San Francisco: Ignatius Press, 2004: pp. 90-95.

Ratzinger, Joseph, "The Dignity of the Human Person" in Herbert Vorgrimler (ed) *Commentary on the Documents of Vatican II* Volume V, London: Burns & Oates, 1969: pp. 115-163.

Rawls, John, *A Theory of Justice*, rev. ed. Cambridge: Belknap Press of Harvard University Press, 1999.

Rawls, John, "The Independence of Moral Theory", *Proceedings and Addresses of the American Philosophical Association*, Vol.47, No.5, p. 22, in *Collected Papers*, 1999: pp. 286-302.

Rawls, John, *Political Liberalism*, New York: Columbia University Press, 1996,

Rawls' John, *Justice as Fairness: A Restatement*, Cambridge: Belknap Press, 2001.

Rawls, John, *A Theory of Justice*, New York: Basic Books, 1974.

Rawls, John, "The Idea of Public Reason Revisited" in John Rawls, *The Law of Peoples*, Cambridge: Harvard University Press, 1999.

Rawls, John, *The Law of Peoples*, Cambridge: Harvard University Press, 1999.

Rivera, Geraldo, *Willowbrook: A Report on How It Is and Why It Doesn't Have to Be That Way*, New York: Random House, 1972.

Rowland, Tracey, *Ratzinger's Faith: The Theology of Pope Benedict XVI"*, Oxford: OUP, 2008.

Savulescu, Julian, "The Present-Aim Theory: A Sub-maximizing Theory of Reasons", *Australasian Journal of Philosophy*, Vol. 76, No. 2: pp. 229-243.

Taylor, Charles, "A Secular Age", Cambridge: Harvard University Press, 2007.

The National Commission for the Protection of Human Subjects of Biomedical and Behavioral Research, *The Belmont Report, Ethical Principles and Guidelines for the Protection of Human Subjects of Research* April 18, 1979.

Thomson, Judith Jarvis, "Killing, Letting Die, and the Trolley Problem", *The Monist*, Vol. 59, 1976: pp. 204-17.

Tonti-Filippini, Nicholas. *Ethics and the Treatment of Infertility*, Melbourne: Holy Name Press, 1983.

Tonti-Filippini, Nicholas. *Human Dignity: Autonomy and Sacredness in the International Human Rights Instruments*, 2001, PhD thesis, Department of Philosophy, The University of Melbourne, http://repository.unimelb.edu.au/10187/1396,

Vatican II, *Gaudium et Spes*, 1965.

Tonti-Filippini, Nicholas "IVF: the role of the technician" in *Persona Veritae Morale*, Citta Nuova Editrice, 1986.

Tonti-Filippini, Nicholas, "Natural Law Tensions", *Ethics Education*, Vol. 16, No. 2, 2010.

United Nations *Universal Declaration on the Human Genome and Human Rights* 1997, http://portal.unesco.org/shs/en/ev.php-URL_ID=1881&URL_DO=DO_TOPIC&URL SECTION=201.html.

Vorgrimler, Herbert (ed) *Commentary on the Documents of Vatican II*, Volume V, London: Burns & Oates, 1969.

Waters, Clara Erskine Clemet, *A Handbook of Legendary and Mythological Art*, first published in 1875, http://www.archive.org/details/ahandbooklegend06wategoog.

Young, Robert, *Personal Autonomy: Beyond Negative and Positive Liberty*, London and Sydney: Croome Helm, 1986.

Index

Abbott, The Hon Tony, 132–133
Anamnesis, 100–103, 109
Andrews, The Hon Kevin, 3
Angioplasty, 1
Aquinas, St Thomas, 49, 53, 58–59, 62–63, 65, 72, 74–76, 79, 81–83, 91, 101, 103–105, 109, 113, 147, 149
Assisted Reproductive Technology, 6, 179–180
Augustine, St Bishop of Hippo, 101–103, 118
Australian Association of Catholic Bioethicists, 6
Australian Bureau of Statistics, 125
Australian Catholic Bishops, 4, 6
Australian Health Ethics Committee, 4, 143, 156, 166
Australian Qualifications Framework, 165–166
Autonomy, 13, 17, 19–20, 22–35, 44, 47, 52, 60–61, 117, 120, 146, 153–154, 156, 158, 160, 170

Beauchamp, Tom L, 19–22, 38, 153–154
Belmont Report, 17, 154
Benedict XVI, Pope, 5–6, 12, 61–62, 145
Beneficence, 11, 17–20, 158
Bergmeier, Mrs., 83, 88
Biggs, John, 168, 172
Bigotry, 13, 118, 125–126, 128, 131–134, 138, 144
Billings, Dr John, 2–3
Bioethics, 1, 17–46, 143–164
Biomedicine, 166–167
Black v. The Commonwealth, 129
Bowie, Norman, 38
Boyle, Joseph M., 90–91, 103

Brain Damaged, 162–165

Campbell, Ray, 3, 89, 105
Capital punishment, 1, 46, 168
Catechism of the Catholic Church, 108
Challenges, 7, 173–178
Charles Curran, 73, 75
Childress, James F, 19–22, 154–155
Christian philosopher, 7, 49, 104, 113, 148
Chronic illness, 10, 23
Churchill, Sir Winston, 41
Clarke, Dr Bernard, 2
Comfort, Nathaniel, 40
Commandments, The Ten, 69, 108
Commercialization of Human Tissue, 6
Community of Christ's faithful, 11, 15
Congregation for the Doctrine of the Faith, 3, 47, 49
Conjugality, 67, 114
Conscience, 55, 69, 71, 101–102, 127, 132, 135–136, 141, 174
Constructive Critical Evaluation, 165–181
Constructivism, 167–169, 178
Convention on the Rights of People with Disabilities, 24
Cooper, Dr Adam, 5
Cooperation in evil, 1
Corinthians, 56–57
Coronary disease, 1
Craniotomy, 89–91, 94
Critical Evaluation, 165–178
Culture of death 10-12

Daly SJ, Rev Dr Tom, 2
Decalogue, 39, 54, 76, 84, 98–99, 108, 110

Democracy, 13, 140–141, 154, 166
Department of Philosophy, 4, 6, 60
Deus Caritas Est, 12
Dialogue, 48, 75, 113, 119, 129, 147, 156, 182
Dichotomy, 61, 148
Dignitas Personae, 49, 54, 63, 68, 115
Direct and indirect intention, 88
Disability, 13, 22–24, 33–34, 38, 40, 42, 121, 182
Donum Vitae, 3
Double effect, 71
Double effect reasoning, 72–97
Dworkin, Ronald, 106, 130

Education, 4–5, 25, 30–31, 33, 55, 112, 129, 136–138, 165, 175
Egan, Winifred, 3
Ellington, James W, 26
Elliott, Bishop Peter, 5
Emanuel, Linda L., 71
Engber-Perdersen, Troels, 56, 58
Ephesians, 57
Epistemology, 154
Ethical Guidelines, 6, 17, 54, 153, 157–159, 160–161, 179–181
Ethical guidelines on the use of assisted reproductive technology in clinical practice and research, 179–180
Eugenics, 40–41
European Commission, 125
Euthanasia, 23, 25–26, 30–31, 40, 42–43, 71, 169, 171
Evangelisation, 100, 114–115
Evangelium Vitae, 12, 80, 84–85, 87, 95, 100
Experimenting, 169–173
Eyster, Zachary C, 72

Faculty of Medicine, 4, 6
Faith and Reason, 52, 60–61, 146
Fides et Ratio, 60–61, 146
Finnis, John M., 4, 90
Fisher OP, Bishop Anthony, 3–4, 6

Fitzgerald OP, Rev Fr Laurence, 2
Fitzmeyer SJ, Joseph A., 56
Fleming, Rev Dr John, 3, 126, 129
Fletcher, Joseph, 69–73, 83
Foot, Philippa, 76–77
Ford SDB, Rev Dr Norman, 2
Fox, Renee C, 168–169
Freedom, 24–26, 28, 30–32, 58, 60, 88, 97–99, 107, 112, 123, 127–129, 134–141, 144, 180
Friendship, 10–11, 97–98, 106
Fuchs, Joseph, 72–73, 97
Fundamental Option, 65, 72, 97–99

Galatians, 56, 58
Gamaliel, 56
Gatekeepers, 166–167
Gaudium et Spes, 51–52, 147
Genesis, 7
Gentiles, 55–56
German Federal Department of Health and Welfare, 4, 143
Gospel of life, 10
Government, 3, 5, 11, 30, 54, 66, 123, 125, 127, 129–132, 143–144, 153, 156–157, 159, 164, 166–167
Grace, 6, 48–49, 58, 66, 97, 99–101, 126
Grisez, Germain, 66–67, 86, 89–90, 98–99, 103, 105, 113

Hare, Richard M, 37, 176
Harman, Rev Dr Francis, 2
Hart, Archbishop Denis, 5–6
Health Professionals, 22, 24, 119–121, 141, 160, 162, 167–169, 174
Hearts, 11, 55, 100–101, 109
Hedonism, 35–36
Hellenization, 55–56
Herman, Barbara, 27
Hill, Thomas E. Jnr, 27
Hitler, Adolf, 42
Hogan, Michael, 130–131
Holiness, 107
Holman RSC, Sr Rose, 2

Hoyt, Robert, 74
Human dignity, 9–10, 23, 44, 60, 128, 144, 160, 162
Human flourishing, 10, 25, 112, 181
Human genome, 173
Human nature, 12, 32, 49, 56, 62–63, 68, 101, 103, 105, 112, 115, 150–151, 155
Human person, 1, 11, 50, 52, 60, 105, 107–109, 114, 117, 145, 147, 150, 153, 178
Human research, 156, 158, 164, 167
Human rights, 7, 13, 43–45, 60, 123, 134, 136–139, 155, 173

Illness, 1–2, 4, 42, 121, 151
Imago dei, 7, 63, 109, 144, 150
Inalienable rights, 9, 13, 43, 60, 128
Inherent dignity, 7, 9, 13, 43, 60, 128
Innocent, 73, 77–78, 84, 87–88, 133
Intent, 86, 91–92
International Association of Catholic Bioethicists, 6
International Covenant on Civil and Political Rights, 44, 60, 144, 155
International Covenants on Economic, Social and Cultural Rights, 44
International Theological Commission, 47–48, 53
Intolerance, 13, 123, 125, 136, 138

John Paul II Institute for Marriage and Family, 4, 7, 57, 89
John, Brian and Myrna, 3
Journet, Charles, 128
Justice, 12, 15, 18–20, 37, 55, 60, 70, 75, 84, 106, 114, 116–117, 120, 129, 149, 151, 154, 158, 162, 176
Justice as Fairness, 37
Justification, 19–20, 30, 61, 104–106, 146, 148–149, 151

Kant, Immanuel, 26, 117, 127
Kerr, Fergus, 152

Killing, 43, 73, 75, 77–78, 80–82, 84–85, 87–90, 92–93, 95, 133
Kirsner, Angela, 5
Knauer, Peter, 81–82, 85–87
Knight Commander of St Gregory the Great, 6
Knight of Magistral Grace in Obedience, 6
Krohn, Anna (nee Duffy), 3, 5

Leo XIII, Pope, 58
Letting Die, 78
Liberalism, 24, 27–28, 37, 137
Libertas Praestantissimum, 58
Liberty, 27–30, 33, 52, 137, 163
Life, respect for, 14, 23, 51, 134
Little, Archbishop Sir Frank, 2

MacIntyre, Alasdair, 61–62, 104, 148, 151–153
Manning, Monsignor Kevin (later Bishop of Parramatta), 5
Maritain, 155
May, William E., 75
McCormick, Richard, 73–75, 77–78, 84–87, 89, 91, 95
McMullen, Dr Gabrielle, 2
Mental Deficiency Act, 41
Mercy death 42–43
Metaphysics, 26, 154
Mill, John Stuart, 28, 36, 127
Minimally Responsive State, 161
Minister for Health, 132
Miscarriage, 87
Mitchell, Alex, 131–132
Modes of responsibility, 110–112
Monash University, 2–4, 6, 138
Moral evil, 10, 72, 82, 84–86, 91
Moral Language, 153, 163–165
Moral Relativism, 104
Moral Theologians, 75
Moral Theory, 27, 35, 90, 106, 168
Motherhood, 1, 11
Mulieres Dignitatem, 57

National Catholic Reporter, 74
National Commission for the Protection of Human Subjects of Biomedical and Behavioral Research, 154
National Health and Medical Research Council, 143, 153, 156, 160–161, 167, 179
National Institutes of Health, 17
National Statement on Ethical Conduct in Human Research, 156, 158
Natural Law, 47–51, 53, 55–56, 58–59, 63, 65–66, 82, 100–101, 103–105, 108–110, 112–115, 154
Nazi, 41–44
Neutrality, 123, 128, 130–131
New natural law, 66, 103–104, 113
Nikzor Project, The, 43
Novak, M., 155
Nuremberg, 42

O'Malley, John W., 175
O'Shea, Dr Gerard, 5
Object of the act, 64–65, 77, 80–81, 85, 87, 96
Order of Malta, 6, 11
Organ and Tissue Donation after Death, 160
Organ and Tissue Donation by Living Donors, 160
Organ and Tissue Transplantation, 6, 159–161

Papal Commission on Birth Control, 69, 74, 81
Participation in the Public Square, 134–135
Partnership, 15, 60–68
Pauline principle, 35, 48–49, 53–54, 64–66, 100, 148, 153, 163
Pell, George Cardinal, 138
Personal Autonomy, 156
Pharisaic, 56
Philippians, 58

Physical acts, 82, 84–85, 90
Pius XII, Pope, 69
Pluralism, 104, 126, 138
Pluralist Society, 14, 44, 61–62, 123–124, 126–128, 135, 144, 147
Political Liberalism, 37
Porter, Jean, 90
Post Coma Unresponsiveness, 160
Practicable reasonableness, 108
Preference utilitarianism, 36–37, 176
Prime Minister, 4, 41
Principlism, 17–24, 153–154
Problem, 11, 22, 31, 37–38, 54, 66, 71, 87, 89, 92–93, 126, 133, 152, 166, 168, 173, 176, 178–181
Proportionalism, 65, 72–97
Prouse, Bishop Christopher, 6
Prudence, 14, 109, 118–119, 121–122
Psychological, 27, 34–35, 86–87, 91–96, 98, 127
Public Debate, 14, 48, 61, 123–124, 126–129, 133–134
Public Reason, 14, 68, 115, 135–136, 143–164
Public Square, 129–130, 133–135

Quaestiones Quodlibetales, 75–76

Rahner S.J., 97–98
Ramsey, Paul, 74, 78, 84
Rationality, 26, 151
Ratzinger, Cardinal Joseph, 59, 145
Rawls, John, 14, 37, 135, 176
Regulations, 145, 154
Religious Freedom, 123, 129, 134–141
Respect for life, 14, 23, 51, 134
Respect for persons, 14, 17, 23, 26, 37, 128, 134
Riordan, Marcia, 5
Rivera, Geraldo, 40
Roosevelt, Eleanor, 43
Rowland, A/Prof Tracey, 5
Rowland, Tracey, 52–53
Russian, 82

Sacredness, 11, 13, 23, 50, 54, 60, 170
Santamaria QC, Joseph, 2
Santamaria, BA, 2
Santamaria, Dr Joseph, 2
Santamaria, John, 2
Savulescu, Julian, 38
School of Medicine, 4
Scripture, 60–61, 84, 99, 104, 108, 120, 133, 146, 148
Seal, Dr Eric, 2
Secular Society, 1, 123–141
Secularism, 11, 13, 47, 67, 100, 114, 123, 125–126, 128, 135–141, 159
Self defence, 74, 79–80, 82–84, 86
Self-integration, 106
Sexuality, 4, 6, 50, 116, 150, 168
Sick, 1, 11, 13, 42–43
Situation Ethics, 65, 69–73, 83
Slavery, 25, 30
Spokes OP, Fr Colin, 3
St Augustine of Hippo, 103, 118
St Paul, 55–58, 100, 109, 129
St Thomas Aquinas, 62, 72, 74–76, 79, 81, 101, 103, 105, 109, 147, 149
State Neutrality, 128–131
Stoic, 55–58, 110, 113
Summa Theologica, 79, 105
Swazey, Judith P, 166–167
Synderesis, 100–103
Synod, 52

Tang, Catherine, 168, 172
Tasmanian Department of State Development, 4
Taylor, Charles, 117, 124
Teaching and Learning, 5, 165–181
Technology, 1, 3, 6, 44, 49, 51, 73, 125, 143, 167, 179–180
Teleology, 22, 47, 65, 100, 103, 107, 114, 119, 121, 154
Temperance, 14–15, 55, 116, 116–117, 120
The Theology of the Body, 57
Theory of Justice, 37, 176

Thomism, 53
Thomson, Judith Jarvis, 78
Tonti-Filippini Nicholas, 3, 7, 73, 129
Transplantation, 6, 159–160, 166
Treatment of Infertility, 73
Truth, 30–31, 45, 60, 63–64, 76, 85, 100, 102, 104, 107, 112, 118, 127, 133, 146–148, 149

UNESCO, 4, 173
United Nations, 180
Universal Declaration, 137, 155, 173
Universal Ethic, 39, 44, 47–121
Unresponsive State, 6
US Congress, 4, 17, 143
Utilitarianism, 35–39, 72, 153, 176

Vatican Council II, 97–98
Vegetative state, 160
Veritatis Splendor, 54, 64, 80, 91, 95, 99, 107
Victorian Assisted Reproductive Technology Authority, 6
Virtue, 14, 22, 45, 49, 55, 61–63, 65–66, 112, 149, 151, 153–154, 172, 176
Virtue Ethics, 22, 114, 153–154
Vocation, 10, 22–24, 32, 63, 109, 145, 150
Voluntary euthanasia, 30–31

Walsh, Nicholas, 3
Walsh, Dr Mary, 3–4, 7
Walters RSC, Sr Maureen, 2
Waters, Clara Erskine Clemet, 34
Western culture, 67, 114, 151
Willowbrook State School, 40
Wisdom, 14, 55–56, 59–60, 62, 116, 119–120, 145, 149

Y-generation, 175
Young, Robert, 33

www.ingramcontent.com/pod-product-compliance
Ingram Content Group UK Ltd.
Pitfield, Milton Keynes, MK11 3LW, UK
UKHW041302180426
11947UKWH00009B/635